Hyperkinetic Children
A Neuropsychosocial Approach

C. Keith Conners
Karen C. Wells

Volume 7.
Developmental Clinical Psychology and Psychiatry

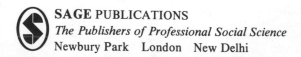

SAGE PUBLICATIONS
The Publishers of Professional Social Science
Newbury Park   London   New Delhi

AAZ2959

This book is dedicated

with loving thanks to

Merle Conners and Annie Laurie Hughes

For information address:

SAGE Publications, Inc.
2111 West Hillcrest Drive
Newbury Park, California 91320

SAGE Publications Ltd.
28 Banner Street
London EC1Y 8QE
England

SAGE Publications India Pvt. Ltd.
M-32 Market
Greater Kailash I
New Delhi 110 048 India

Printed in the United States of America

Library of Congress Cataloging-in-Publication Data

Conners, C. Keith.
  Hyperkinetic children.

  (Developmental clinical psychology and psychiatry
series; v. 7)
    Bibliography: p.
    Includes index.
    1. Hyperactive child syndrome.   2. Neuropsychology.
3. Hyperactive child syndrome—Social aspects.   I. Wells,
Karen C.   II. Title.   III. Series: Developmental clinical
psychology and psychiatry; v. 7.
RJ506.H9C653   1985   618.92′8589   85-19626
ISBN 0-8039-2278-7
ISBN 0-8039-2279-5 (pbk.)

SECOND PRINTING, 1989

SERIES EDITOR'S INTRODUCTION

Interest in child development and adjustment is by no means new. Yet, only recently has the study of children benefited from advances in both clinical and scientific research. Many reasons might explain the recent systematic attention to children, including more pervasive advances in research in the social and biological sciences, the emergence of disciplines and subdisciplines that focus exclusively on childhood and adolescence, and greater appreciation of the impact of such influences as the family, peers, school, and many other factors on child adjustment. Apart from interest in the study of child development and adjustment for its own sake, the need to address clinical problems of adulthood naturally draws one to investigate precursors in childhood and adolescence.

Within a relatively brief period, the study of childhood development, child psychopathology, and child mental health has evolved and proliferated considerably. In fact, several professional journals, annual book series, and handbooks devoted entirely to the study of children and adolescents and their adjustment document the proliferation of work in the field. Although many different disciplines and specialty areas contribute to knowledge of childhood disorders, there is a paucity of resource material that presents information in an authoritative, systematic, and disseminable fashion. There is a need within the field to present the latest developments and to represent different disciplines, multiple approaches to, and conceptual views of the topics of childhood adjustment and maladjustment.

The Sage *Developmental Clinical Psychology and Psychiatry* Series is designed to serve uniquely several needs of the field. The series encompasses individual monographs prepared by experts in the fields of clinical child psychology, child psychiatry, child development, and related disciplines. The primary focus is on childhood psychopathology, which refers broadly here to the diagnosis, assessment, treatment, and prevention of problems of children and adolescents. The scope of the series is necessarily broad because of the working assumption, if not demonstrated fact, that understanding, identifying, and treating problems of youth regrettably cannot be resolved by narrow, single-discipline, and parochial conceptual views. Thus, the series draws upon multiple disciplines and diverse views within a given discipline.

The task for individual contributors is to present the latest theory and research on various topics including specific types of dysfunction, diagnostic and treatment approaches, and special problem areas that affect adjustment. Core topics within child clinical work are addressed by the series. Authors are asked to bridge potential theory and research, research and clinical practice, and current status and future directions. The goals of the series and the tasks presented to individual contributors are demanding. We have been extremely fortunate in recruiting leaders in the fields who have been able to translate their recognized scholarship and expertise into highly readable works on contemporary topics.

Among clinical dysfunctions of childhood, few have received as much attention as hyperactivity or hyperkinesis. Many books have been written on the topic and a great deal of research continues to be reported. The present book, *Hyperkinetic Children: A Neuropsychosocial Approach,* integrates historical and contemporary research on the nature of the dysfunction and its characteristics. In this book, Drs. C. Keith Conners and Karen C. Wells make a unique contribution by advancing a position that integrates neuropsychological functioning and socioenvironmental influences in accounting for the characteristics of hyperkinesis. Yet, the book was not written to advance a particular view but rather to incorporate what is known about the dysfunction, its diagnosis, assessment, and treatment. The product is a book that is guided by a conceptual position and that relies heavily upon current empirical research. Key topics are addressed including the role of attentional problems and motor activity in the dysfunction and response to stimulant medication and the role of multiple treatments in short- and long-term course of the dysfunction. The topic of hyperkinesis is one to which the contributions of the authors are already well known. The present book provides a comprehensive, integrative, and strongly empirical addition that yields an important substantive advance.

—*Alan E. Kazdin, Ph.D.*
Series Editor

PREFACE

Hyperkinesis in children has been a focus of controversy for over three decades. This book asks why this controversy has led to so many facts but so little understanding. We believe that the basic phenomena, described so concisely by Laufer and Denhoff, who coined the term "hyperkinetic behavior syndrome" many years ago, can best be understood from the perspective of the way the brain is organized, develops over time, and interacts with the environment. Our argument, then, is fundamentally neuropsychological.

The concept of hyperkinetic behavior syndrome was proposed in its original form as a manifestation of brain dysfunction. Since the syndrome was first proposed, however, new methods and concepts of brain organization and function have become available, considerably broadening our understanding of brain-behavior relationships. We have tried to integrate some of this newer understanding from neuroanatomy and neurophysiology of the brain with the basic clinical phenomena.

It has often been said that 90% of the brain is engaged in controlling the actions of the other 10%. We argue that the primary symptoms of hyperkinesis reflect this interplay between brain mechanisms that incite to action on the one hand and inhibit it on the other. But dysfunctions in these systems produce strikingly different patterns of behavior among individual patients, partly because the higher-order systems are themselves composed of intricate subsystems, and partly because the brain is an open system whose very structure feeds upon the environment that nurtures it. Symptoms can only provide a fuzzy and approximate view into the many disturbances to which the brain is heir during its evolution and development.

This book represents an extended argument that there is both unity and diversity in the symptoms of the hyperkinetic child. When painted in the broad strokes of the clinician, one readily identifies children who fit the concept of a "syndrome" of hyperkinesis. But when examined more closely using tools that reflect subtleties of brain function, the apparent syndrome dissolves into distinguishable subtypes that have a different response to treatment, different patterning of symptoms, and different life courses.

This book is addressed to graduate students and researchers of childhood psychopathology who are confronted with opposing views that state that hyperkinesis is either myth or reality, either a meaningless hodgepodge of brat behaviors or a medical syndrome, and who are understandably confused by the plethora of theories and empirical data that have turned the topic into a cottage industry for a generation of researchers and clinicians. We are under no illusion that our views will be readily accepted, but hope that by emphasizing the conceptual aspects of the problem a more productive dialogue will ensue.

We are indebted to a small core of research teams who have diligently applied their efforts and made original observations over the years, including Maurice Laufer and Eric Denhoff; John Peters, Sam Clements and Roscoe Dykman; John Werry, Gabrielle Weiss and Lily Hechtman; Jan Loney; Rachel Gittelman; Russell Barkley; Dennis Cantwell and James Satterfield; Carol Whalen and Barbara Henker; Robert Sprague and Esther Sleator; Judith Rapoport; Michael Rutter and Eric Taylor; and to our mentors Leon Eisenberg and Rex Forehand for their support and guidance early in our careers.

We are particularly grateful to Ronald Lipman who almost singlehandedly shaped the progress of the field by his continuing efforts to enlist qualified researchers into the field of pediatric psychopharmacology, from which much of the relevant research has emerged. We are grateful to our Chairman, James Egan, M.D., for encouraging us in our research and allowing us the freedom to arrange our schedules in the interest of this project.

—*C. Keith Conners*
Karen C. Wells

1

WHAT IS HYPERKINESIS?

Hyperactivity is unique among the childhood behavior disorders in that
the whole field is characterized to an unusual degree by uncertainty,
contradictions, the unexpected, and the bizarre.

—Ross and Ross (1982, p. 6)

In 1854 the German physician Hoffman described in humorous
doggerel a mischievous, impulsive, troublesome youngster by the name
of Fidgety Phil. It has been suggested that perhaps hyperkinesis should
be named "Hoffman's disease" (Cantwell, 1984). But is hyperkinesis[1] a
disease or merely the normally bothersome behavior of an undisciplined
and unruly child? Is it a syndrome, or an unrelated set of complaints tied
together only by the fact that a parent or teacher is annoyed with the
child? Widely divergent opinions are found in the literature. When a
question such as the title of this chapter persists unanswered for so long,
perhaps it is time to review the way the questions have been asked rather
than continue piling up more facts in answer to old questions. We begin,
then, with expert opinions regarding the syndrome, to see in what
manner the questions have been posed.

EXPERT OPINIONS

Laufer and Denhoff

The first systematic description of the hyperkinetic syndrome was
given by Maurice Laufer, a child psychiatrist, and Eric Denhoff, a pe

11

diatric neurologist (Laufer & Denhoff, 1957). Their characterization of the disorder reflects the influence of their disciplines. In addition to viewing the disorder as a medical syndrome, they suggested a specific pathophysiological mechanism to account for the major symptoms, psychological mechanisms to account for the minor symptoms, and a multifaceted therapeutic regimen which included medication, education, and psychotherapy. (Ironically, and somewhat prophetically, they hoped that the success of stimulant medication would not lead to indiscriminate drug treatment and the neglect of psychotherapy.)

As described by Laufer and Denhoff, the essential symptoms of the disorder consist of hyperactivity, short attention span and poor powers of concentration, variability in performance and behavior, impulsiveness and inability to delay gratification, irritability, explosiveness, and poor school work. School difficulties were viewed as a consequence of the conduct disturbances as well as "a compound of problems in the visuo-motor-perception and concentration areas" (1957, p. 464).

All of these primary symptoms are viewed as a direct consequence of a defect in the diencephalon of the brain. The diencephalon is a complex set of subcortical structures which includes the thalamus, hypothalamus, subthalamus, and epithalamus. These structures serve many functions, including that of a relay station for the transmission of information regarding sensation and movement as well as homeostatic (hypothalamic) functions influencing endocrine control via the anterior and posterior pituitary gland. Also of importance are the connections from diencephalic structures to a ring of cortical structures referred to as the limbic system, which regulates emotional expression and response. Laufer and Denhoff believed that any number of different causes might lead to subcortical damage, with the resultant symptom picture depending upon what other brain areas were also implicated. Thus, these authors believed that the hyperkinetic syndrome was due to a single core defect that leads to "an undue sensitivity of the central nervous system to stimuli constantly pouring in from peripheral receptors and from viscera" (1957, p. 467).

Although these authors believed that brain dysfunction lay at the root of the disorder, they were careful to point out that *brain injury* is by no means characteristic of the disorder. Many of the children they studied were seen at the Emma Pendleton Bradley Home, an inpatient residential facility in which many postencephalitic, epileptic and brain-injured children resided. Although the syndrome was associated with cerebral palsy in 23% of the cases, the various consequences of brain injury could occur independently of the hyperkinetic syndrome. The authors stated quite explicitly that there were many different consequences of injury to the brain, depending upon the locus, type, and timing of the insult; these other patterns of brain injury were carefully distinguished from the hyperkinetic syndrome that was thought to be the specific result of dysfunction or damage in the diencephalon.

They made important observations concerning the developmental course of the disorder. Developmental histories frequently reveal a child who climbed out of the crib well before a year of age, walked early, and after that "there was no holding him." However, the hyperactivity may first appear anywhere up to 6 years of age, often becoming noticeable only when the child first enters school. Parents of these older children frequently remark that the child is always on the go and frequently is unable to sit still even to eat or stay in line for assembly in school.

The age at which a diagnosis can be made is complicated by the variability in the time of appearance of the behavioral signs. One or more of the primary symptoms may become the focus of parental concerns. But the other primary symptoms will generally be detectable upon close scrutiny. In infancy there may be excessive irritability and readiness to cry, or unusual placidity, an advanced developmental schedule, and exceedingly active behavior of all kinds. Sleep disturbances are common and consist of difficulty falling asleep, or more often falling asleep at the normal time but wakening after a few hours, often followed by vocalizing in bed or rampaging through the house in innocent but aggravating play.

Laufer and Denhoff believed that a number of secondary symptoms occur in these children because of their unusual sensitivity to internal and external stimuli. So-called colic—querulousness, irritability, squirming, tenseness, demanding and unsatisfied behavior—reflects the infant's greater vulnerability to otherwise normal visceral and appetitive stimuli. Flooded with tension, the infant reacts in a manner similar to children who undergo severe privation or hospitalism. A parallel is drawn with the stimulus-hungry orphan "a bottomless over-demanding, and never-satisfied pit of insatiable wants and requirements" (1957, p. 465). The child with a diencephalic dysfunction is unable to modulate or screen out stimuli from peripheral or visceral receptors. Such a child often succeeds in gradually creating a mother who doubts her own worth and eventually builds up a reservoir of hostility toward the child, setting off a train of emotional disturbances in both the parent and the child. This transaction between biological and social forces thus accounts for much of the secondary pathology.

Hyperkinesis does not protect the child against neuroses, but on the contrary predisposes to them. Although quite independently the child may develop classic neurotic patterns such as anxiety reactions, phobias, obsessions, and compulsions, most of the neurotic disturbances were seen by these authors as the "acting out" variety, such as lying, stealing, assault, truancy, excessive eating, and destructiveness. The child's weaknesses in perception, motor control, and ability to inhibit and redirect impulses and to withstand stresses leads to a variety of school difficulties as well as a distorted and unfavorable self-image and unhappiness. Many symptoms that others might consider evidence of a primary conduct disorder, these authors viewed as secondary neurotic or learned consequences of the neurologically vulnerable child. They were certainly aware that lying, stealing and truanting could be symptoms of an entirely different disorder, but might also be the learned consequences of a fundamental hyperkinetic impulse disorder.

The diagnosis of the syndrome is made primarily from history. The standard neurological examination seldom provides useful information, though failure to copy geometric figures is one of the most consistent and helpful signs of the condition. Psychological test performances usually associated with brain dysfunction occur, but usually with a lack of consistency of such findings within the total battery. When such signs do appear, they are thought to reflect a combination of perceptual-motor immaturity, or impulsivity in thinking and action.

Minimal Brain Dysfunction

Although many early workers in the field were impressed with the variety of behavioral disturbances which followed known brain insults, such as viral encephalitis and head injury, the concept of a behavior disorder resulting from brain damage gradually gave way to a more subtle concept of brain dysfunction which had an important impact upon treatment, education, and diagnosis. Kessler (1980) provides a detailed account of this development. It was Herbert Birch (1964) who most clearly insisted on the distinction between brain damage as a *fact* in contradistinction to the *hypothesis* of brain dysfunction.

The transition from damage to dysfunction was formalized by a government-sponsored task force under the direction of Clements (1966). This influential report had much to do with the emergence of the concept of "minimal brain dysfunction" (MBD), essentially an alternative name for the hyperkinetic syndrome but including other symptom patterns as well. This much-quoted definition stated,

The term "minimal brain dysfunction" refers in this paper to children of near average, average or above average general intelligence with certain learning or behavioral disabilities ranging from mild to severe, which are associated with deviations of functions of the central nervous system. These deviations may manifest themselves by various combinations of impairment in perception, conceptualization, language, memory, and control of attention, impulse, or motor function. (1966, p. 9)

With admirable clarity the author of this report recognized that manifestations of central nervous system (CNS) dysfunctions can be inferred only from various combinations of impairment in perceptual, conceptual, linguistic, mnestic, attentional, or motor functions. There is no implication that all manifestations of impairment reflect CNS dysfunctions; it is patterns of symptoms that differentiate organic from nonorganic disturbances. In large part this statement was meant to counterbalance the one-sided, often fanciful psychodynamic explanations frequently given for any deviant child behavior (Kessler, 1980).

The American Psychiatric Association

In its second edition of its Diagnostic and Statistical Manual (DSM-II, 1968), the APA proposed the diagnosis of Hyperkinetic Reaction of Childhood without reference to its organic basis, calling it

a disorder characterized by overactivity, restlessness, distractibility, and short attention span, especially in young children; the behavior usually diminishes in adolescence.

Hyperkinesis is seen here as essentially a developmental phenomenon, a disorder that begins early in life and wanes with adolescence.

Whereas Laufer and Denhoff had posited seven primary symptoms of the disorder, tied together by a common etiology, and Clements had emphasized a wide range of possible symptomatic deviations, the evolution of thinking over the 12 years between the second and third edition of the APA Diagnostic Manual resulted in a focus on attentional disturbances, with hyperactivity no longer a primary symptom at all. Thus, according to this most recent formula, in DSM-III hyperactivity is not an independent syndrome, but merely an associated feature of an attentional deficit syndrome (Table 1.1).

This rather dramatic shift in emphasis was influenced by a large number of studies that, in one way or another, implicated disturbance of attention as a distinguishing feature between hyperactive and nonhy-

TABLE 1.1

Diagnostic Criteria for Attention Deficit Disorder (ADD) with Hyperactivity

The child displays, for his or her mental and chronological age, signs of developmentally inappropriate inattention, impulsivity, and hyperactivity. The signs must be reported by adults in the child's environment, such as parents and teachers. Because the symptoms are typically variable, they may not be observed directly by the clinician. When the reports of teachers and parents conflict, primary consideration should be given to the teacher reports because of greater familiarity with age–appropriate norms. Symptoms typically worsen in situations that require self-application, as in the classroom. Signs of the disorder may be absent when the child is in a new or a one-to-one situation.

The number of symptoms specified is for children between the ages of 8 and 10, the peak age for referral. In younger children, more severe forms of the symptoms and a greater number of symptoms are usually present. The opposite is true of older children.

A. *Inattention.* At least three of the following:
(1)   often fails to finish things he or she starts,
(2)   often doesn't seem to listen,
(3)   easily distracted,
(4)   has difficulty concentrating on schoolwork or other tasks requiring sustained attention,
(5)   has difficulty sticking to a play activity.

B. *Impulsivity.* At least three of the following:
(1)   often acts before thinking,
(2)   shifts excessively from one activity to another,
(3)   has difficulty organizing work (this not being due to cognitive impairment),
(4)   needs a lot of supervision,
(5)   frequently calls out in class,
(6)   has difficulty awaiting turn in games or group situations.

C. *Hyperactivity.* At least two of the following:
(1)   runs about or climbs on things excessively,
(2)   has difficulty sitting still or fidgets excessively,
(3)   has difficulty staying seated,
(4)   moves about excessively during sleep,
(5)   is always "on the go" or acts as if "driven by a motor."

D. Onset before the age of 7.

E. Duration of a least 6 months.

F. Not due to Schizophrenia, Affective Disorder, or Severe or Profound Mental Retardation.

SOURCE: From the *Diagnostic and Statistical Manual of Mental Disorders* (3rd ed.). Washington, DC: American Psychiatric Association, 1980. Copyright 1980 by the American Psychiatric Association. Reprinted by permission.

peractive children (Douglas & Peters, 1979), and the failure of other proposed syndrome measures to agree or to consistently differentiate hyperactive from nonhyperactive samples (Routh & Roberts, 1972). The developers of DSM-III also felt that although attention may not be the core symptom of the syndrome, it may be more important than activity level; and impulsivity may be equally important. Finally, they recognized that some children have attentional disturbances without the other problems, and that adolescents and adults may continue to manifest attentional problems and impulse control problems without being motorically overactive (Cantwell, 1983).

While reasonable on the face of it, this approach seems quite anomalous in another respect: Most of the research studies that found attentional dysfunctions in hyperactive compared to nonhyperactive samples *first classified them on the basis of a clinical or rating method heavily influenced by behavioral hyperactivity.*

Thus, the finding of objectively measured attentional disturbance in hyperactive children must mean that they have both attentional and activity level dysfunctions. Inconsistency in the discriminative power of objective motor behavior measures can only mean that these more "objective" indices of activity level have low correlations with the original symptomatic measure of activity level upon which the diagnosis was based. We will examine this issue further in the following chapter.

Looking at the DSM-III definitions of inattention and hyperactivity as primary symptoms, it is also obvious that the two are operationally the same: There is no way a child can "finish things he starts" and also be "constantly on the go." Running about is an incompatible response with concentrating on schoolwork. It seems most likely, then, that samples selected using the DSM-III diagnosis must, perforce, be both attentionally and motorically impaired. Particularly when the samples are defined by observer judgments of "always on the go" or "can't sit still," one would expect that the children would also be characterized as showing "difficulty concentrating" or "sticking to a task." What is most important, however, is that DSM-III appears to have implicitly adopted the position that independent dimensions may coalesce in particular children so as to produce a child with a "disorder."

In addition to these formal attempts to characterize the syndrome, a number of clinicians and scholars have attempted to synthesize available research investigations. How have they viewed the definition of hyperkinesis?

Dennis Cantwell

Dennis Cantwell was one of the psychiatrists responsible for attempting to bring a more rigorous and operational definition of the hyperactivity syndrome into psychiatric practice. He describes the clinical picture of the hyperactive child syndrome as varying

> from the little boy who is silly, immature and not performing academically up to expected standards to the markedly active, aggressive and antisocial child who is unable to be managed in a regular classroom setting. (Cantwell, 1975, p. 5)

He considers the syndrome to consist of the cardinal symptoms of hyperactivity, distractibility, impulsivity, excitability, antisocial behavior, and cognitive and learning disabilities. Symptoms often associated with the syndrome are aggressive and antisocial behavior, cognitive and learning disabilities, and emotional symptoms such as depression and low self-esteem. One of the features of Cantwell's approach is the willingness to consider that there may be distinctive subtypes of the disorder. For example, there may be genetically different subtypes depending upon whether the families have a genetic loading for the disorder.

In two important studies Cantwell (1972) and Morrison and Stewart (1971) showed that the hyperactive child syndrome was found to a much greater degree in the biologic first- and second-degree relatives of hyperactive children than in the relatives of adopted hyperactive children. An increased rate of alcoholism, sociopathy, and hysteria were found in the biologic but not the adoptive parents of hyperactive children. Methodologically these studies suffer from a lack of blind assessment of the index groups, and a failure to interview the biologic parents of adopted hyperactive children. But the available data are certainly consistent with the hypothesis that there is at least one subtype which is genetic in origin.

Cantwell also considers the possibility that there may be distinctive subgroups based upon neurologic dysfunction, abnormalities in the electroencephalogram (EEG), and patterns of antisocial and aggressive behavior. Despite a description of the syndrome in purely behavioral terms, Cantwell's *conceptualization* of the problem is unabashedly aligned with a "medical model" approach for integrating aspects of the clinical picture. Often used as a term of abuse, Cantwell states that the medical model approach is heuristically useful. This approach follows suggestions by Guze (1970) and Robins and Guze (1970) that (1) child psychiatry is a branch of medicine; (2) focus is on a condition, disorder, or disease; (3) patients may present with many types of disorders differing in pathogenesis, etiology, symptomatology, natural history, and response to treatment; and (4) precisely defined diagnostic categories are required for advancement in the field.

Safer and Allen

Safer and Allen (1976) reject the position that hyperactivity is a syndrome on the one hand, or that it is a useless wastebasket of symptoms on the other. Instead, they restrict the terminology of the hyperactive child to the "persistent pattern of excessive activity in situations requiring motor inhibition" (1976, p. 7). In addition, they ascribe inattentiveness, learning impediments, behavior problems, and immaturity as major features of the disorder, while minor features include impulsivity, peer difficulties, and low self-esteem. They believe that hyperactivity, the core symptom, is developmental in nature and occurs in early childhood, even though it is often most strikingly revealed in the classroom in later childhood.

As in the original description by Laufer and Denhoff, Safer and Allen find support for the diagnosis from abnormal Bender-Gestalt drawings, nonspecific EEG abnormality, pediatric neurologic examination, IQ testing (which tends to be about 10 points lower than children from the same neighborhood), and academic testing. They take the position that although developmental hyperactivity is not a true diagnostic syndrome, it is nevertheless specific enough to provide useful guidance in treatment and prognosis.

Although these authors eschew a firm commitment to an organic etiology, the fact that one-third of hyperactive children are learning-impaired, one-tenth have a history of seizures, one-half have abnormal EEGs, and one-third to one-half have signs of neurological delays make the conclusion of an organic etiology "hard to resist" (1976, p. 29).

John Werry

Werry (1979) finds that although the diagnostic entity of hyperkinetic syndrome is controversial, clinically diagnosed hyperactive children, as a group, are clearly differentiated from normal and from anxious-withdrawn children, with the primary symptoms showing "a remarkable consistency across different observers" (1979, p. 112).

Werry also finds that the research literature provides support for the role of noxious insults to the brain, soft neurological abnormalities, mild abnormalities of cognition and perception, mild EEG abnormalities, sensorimotor incoordination, and minor physical anomalies. Like Cantwell, Werry suggests that further subclassifications of the syndrome based upon multivariate approaches to clinical, neurological, and psychophysiological data will be required before issues of etiological explanation can be resolved.

Carol Whalen

In a series of original empirical and theoretical papers Whalen and her colleagues have explored the role of social system and institutional contexts in defining, measuring, and treating hyperactive children (Whalen & Henker, 1976; Whalen & Henker, 1977; Whalen & Henker, 1980a, 1980b; Whalen, Collins, Henker, Alkus, Adams, & Stapp, 1978; Whalen, Henker, Collins, Finck, & Dotemoto 1979a; Whalen, Henker, Collins, McAuliffe, & Vaux, 1979b; Whalen, Henker & Dotemoto, 1981; Whalen, Henker & Finck, 1981; Whalen, 1983).

Regarding diagnosis, Whalen states that

> the pattern of dysfunctional behaviors differs from child to child, and may result from diverse and complexly interactive biological and psychological processes. In other words, the key feature is heterogeneity—in the children, the behavior patterns and concomitants, the probable causes, and the likely outcomes. (1983, p. 159)

Whalen sees the diagnostic terms hyperactivity and hyperkinesis as convenient descriptive terms referring "to a large group of children who have *serious* difficulties concentrating, inhibiting inappropriate responses, and getting along in the everyday world" (1983, p. 153). Reviewing problem domains of attention, cognition and learning, motoric activity, and social competence, Whalen concludes that there is little consistency demonstrating covariance either across or within domains; that hyperactive children are not consistently characterized as inattentive, motorically disinhibited, dysfunctional in cognition or social behaviors; and within a single domain there are no consistent indicators of dysfunction such as a uniform deficit in particular measures of attention.

Perhaps the most original contribution of these investigators has been the demonstration of child by situation interactions. Rather than viewing hyperactivity as either a deficit in the child or as environmentally caused, these investigators demonstrate that variations in classroom dimensions, such as ambient noise, task difficulty, and degree of externally imposed structure amplify or diminish differences between hyperactive and normal children. Social communication patterns, noise-making and disruption vary as a function of both the child's status (normal versus hyperactive) and environmental constraints.[2]

Russell Barkley

With uncompromising thoroughness, Barkley reviewed over 200 studies of hyperactive children and found that more than 70% failed to use any objective or specifiable criteria for diagnosing children as hyperactive, "other than the mere opinion of the author of the study" (Barkley, 1981, p. 4). Barkley criticizes the DSM-III version of Attention Deficit Disorder (ADD) for several reasons: first for making a distinction of ADD with and without hyperactivity as being unfounded; for ignoring the issue of pervasiveness of the symptoms; for ignoring the criteria for severity; for arbitrarily setting the age of onset criterion as less than age 7; and, finally, for failing to specify how one should determine whether the child's symptoms are age-inappropriate.

Barkley also made an important additional distinction based upon work (Barkley & Cunningham, 1979; Campbell, 1975) that showed that hyperactive children are less compliant, more attention seeking, and more in need of supervision than normal children. He proposed that what was seen as a secondary symptom by Laufer and Denhoff be regarded as a primary or essential symptom:

> Hyperactivity is a developmental disorder of age-appropriate attention span, impulse control, restlessness, and rule-governed behavior that develops in late infancy or early childhood (before age 6), is pervasive in nature, and is not accounted for on the basis of gross neurologic, sensory, or motor impairment, or severe emotional disturbance. (Barkley, 1981, p. 6)

Barkley's studies of family interactions among hyperactives led him to place more emphasis than previously upon noncompliance or "rule-governed behavior." Barkley's rationale for considering noncompliance as a separate criterion is that it shows a good correlation with rating scale measures of hyperactivity and low correlations with measures of activity level or attention span.[3]

The suggestion that noncompliance is a failure of rule-governed behavior now places this concept close to traditional concepts of conduct disorder, a condition of "not following the rules" par excellence. However, since Barkley also believes that conduct disorder should be separated from hyperkinesis per se (1981), he appears to be suggesting a different theoretical construct of conduct disorder, having to do with the failure to acquire rules and to self-regulate behavior. In his discussion of this topic Barkley (1981) links the concept to Luria's notion of self-directed speech as a basis for sustaining attention and impulse, and cites the fact that high-activity children who have mature language development are less likely to make impulsive errors on a visual matching task than high-activity children with immature language development. By implication, Barkley appears to be suggesting a form of conduct disorder involving higher-order self-regulation as distinguished, perhaps, from a purely environmentally determined or learned form of the disorder.

Barkley also concludes that hyperactivity is not a syndrome, basing his argument upon the failure of measures of activity level, attention span, and impulsivity to covary uniformly in hyperactive children. "The conclusion has been that hyperactivity comprises a quite heterogeneous group of children, with some being inattentive, others being overactive, and still others having both symptoms" (1981, p. 15). Consistent with this approach is the opinion that no single etiology for the disorder can be found.

Ross and Ross

Unquestionably the most comprehensive, balanced and scholarly account of hyperactivity as a behavior disorder is provided by Ross and Ross (1982). Their bibliography of over 1,000 references attests to both their scholarly commitment and the extent of the verbiage poured out on this topic. They conceptualized hyperactivity as

> a class of heterogeneous behavior disorders in which a high level of activity that is exhibited at inappropriate times and cannot be inhibited upon command is often the major presenting complaint. (1982, p. 14)

This definition is somewhat different than many others; it requires a high level of *inappropriate activity,* and a failure of *voluntary inhibition.* Some or all of a number of other symptoms may be present: hyperactivity, short attention span, distractibility, impulsivity, emotional liability, low frustration tolerance, aggressiveness, destructiveness, poor school performance, and poor peer relationships.

Ross and Ross also find that hyperactivity is not a syndrome. Reasons given for this finding are that factor analytic studies fail to define a unitary cluster of characteristics, the lack of a common cause and a consistent response to treatment, and a lack of consistent differences between hyperactivity and other disorders, particularly conduct disorders. They conclude that there may be several hyperactivity syndromes, not a single entity that qualifies as a homogeneous disorder.

Michael Rutter

Many of the same arguments against hyperactivity as a syndrome have been put forth by Rutter (1982, 1983). First, Rutter (1982) notes that studies have shown low levels of agreement among parents, teachers, and clinicians on the diagnosis (Kenny et al., 1971; Lambert, Sandoval, & Sassone, 1978). Low levels of agreement among professionals is supported by findings that the syndrome is diagnosed 50 times more often in North America than in Great Britain (Rutter, Shaffer & Shepherd, 1975) despite a similar factor structure and distribution of symptoms in the two areas (Sandberg, Weiselberg & Shaffer, 1980).

Second, several measurement issues are raised by Rutter. Different measures of hyperactivity intercorrelate quite weakly; no overall factor of hyperactivity is found, but rather factors reflecting the source of the information (Langhorne, Loney, Paternite, & Bechtoldt, 1976); and finally, questionnaire measures of overactivity correlate highly with measures of general conduct disturbance. Rutter sees the issue of differentiation of a syndrome, with the real issue being whether proposed syndrome characteristics differentiate between hyperactives and other psychiatric conditions.

Rutter further points out that the symptoms of hyperactivity and inattention are themselves not unitary. Fidgeting and squirming are not the same as running about aimlessly. Moreover, different facets of inattention and hyperactivity are differentially responsive to stimulant medication (Conners & Werry, 1979). Finally, Rutter reviews evidence to suggest that *pervasive* hyperactivity may constitute a valid syndrome, whereas situational hyperactivity does not. However, he concludes that this group would be very rare, constituting at most 2% of the usual clinic samples. In a conclusion strikingly similar to other authors we have reviewed, Rutter states that broad, ill-defined groups of restless, disruptive and fidgety children have been lumped under a global concept which conceals real differences among them.

SUMMARY AND CONCLUSIONS

The scholarly opinions we have reviewed share important similarities in conceptualization of hyperkinesis. The symptoms appear to come from the same pot, but are sometimes stirred a bit differently. The range of symptoms involved seems for the most part to reflect a difference in emphasis rather than fundamental disagreement. Some place the "core" symptoms differently, opting either for attention or activity level; what are secondary symptoms for some are core for others.

The most disagreement is over the status of the concept: Is it a syndrome or something else? Whereas Laufer and Denhoff, Clements, and Cantwell view hyperkinesis as a syndrome, Rutter, Ross and Ross, Barkley, and Werry do not. Safer and Allen come down firmly in the middle of the fence, preferring an intermediate level concept which has treatment and prognostic value without fulfilling criteria for a true syndrome.

Only Laufer and Denhoff were bold enough to speculate about a particular mechanism (diencephalic dysfunction) that could serve as the "final common pathway" in the nervous system through which various insults could express their effect. Almost all of the authors explicitly view the hyperkinetic syndrome as heterogeneous and capable of being refined into subgroups. They share the view that no single etiology can account for the disorder.

What seems to be lacking in all of these integrative expositions is any conceptual model that goes beyond the relatively uninformative and global proposition that genetic, traumatic, temperamental, and environmental causes somehow produce problems in attention, impulse, and activity level. Unfortunately, much of the research has added data without conceptualization to explain the data. Only Laufer and Denhoff provided an explicit account of how the primary symptoms arise, interact with the environment, and progress to secondary symptoms.

Almost all of the work on this issue is confounded by the bootstrap problem: Until one knows how to classify the subjects into homogeneous groups there is no hope of finding either unique biological or environmental causes, to say nothing of the *transactional* causative networks that, in the final analysis, are the most likely explanatory systems for such complex behavioral manifestations. Until one is able to focus in on particular causative pathways there is no hope of selecting the relevant homogeneous samples by which the causal network can be explicated. As pointed out by Eysenck many years ago, taxonomy is a prerequisite to measurement (1952) and as yet, there has not been an adequate classification system for taking the first step of selecting a homogeneous group. While more operational than earlier definitions, DSM-III is somewhat arbitrary in the way the symptom pie is sliced and apportioned to different disorders.

In the following chapter we start with a classification based upon a deliberately broad concept of behavior disorders: externalizing symptomatology versus internalizing symptomatology. Many of the phenomena attributed to the hyperkinetic child can be subsumed under this rubric. But even behavioral symptomatology is more complex than this, and other dimensions will be seen to be at play in the symptom patterns observed in the clinic. There are several different patterns of symptoms among children usually labeled "hyperkinetic."

Using dimensions of symptomatology as a classification or taxonomic device, however, is not sufficient. Many of the same disturbances at a symptomatic level can be caused by quite different underlying brain processes, and for tapping these processes we need methods which are more properly called *neuropsychological*. In subsequent chapters we will explore some of the concepts which have been used to characterize hyperactives, including cognitive, attentional, and motor phenomena. In each case we will point to the multidimensionality of these concepts, and the way various facets of the global concepts interplay to produce recognizable subtypes of hyperkinesis.

NOTES

1. Leo Kanner once noted that it ought to be forbidden to mix Greek prefixes such as "hyper" with Roman suffixes such as "activity." (Certainly no one has been audacious enough to use the construction of "overkinesis".) We usually reserve the term hyperkinesis for the concept of an entity or syndrome, and hyperactivity for a particular kind of symptom. But we confess that etymologic rigor often succumbs to the temptation of common parlance. When we refer to hyperkinetics we usually refer to "him"—not out of sexist bias but because males have the dubious distinction of a 5 or 10 to 1 advantage in numbers with regards to the diagnosis.

2. Similar reasoning led us to examine the interaction of stress and informational load with stimulant drug effects (Conners, 1975a), and structured versus unstructured environments in treatment response (Conners & Wells, 1979).

3. Here again, some circularity in reasoning appears to have crept in: Since Barkley's study samples were largely selected by rating scales that are heavily weighted toward reporting noncompliance, finding this feature as a regular accompaniment of hyperactivity is not surprising.

2

A CLINICAL STUDY OF HYPERKINETIC CHILDREN

"If it's a dichotomy, it's wrong."
—Harry Harlow

THE STUDY

At the time of Laufer and Denhoff's description of the hyperkinetic behavior syndrome, the American Psychiatric Association, like the World Health Organization, distinguished two broad classes of non-organic and nonpsychotic disturbances: conduct disorders and neuroses.

These concepts were evident in the early work in childhood psychopharmacology begun by Bradley (1937, 1950), and continued by Eisenberg and colleagues (Eisenberg, Gilbert, Cytryn, & Molling, 1961; Eisenberg et al., 1963; Cytryn, Gilbert, & Eisenberg, 1960). Samples were selected from children referred for outpatient psychiatric treatment who had IQs above 80, who were not psychotic or organically impaired, and who had no history of clear-cut delinquent behavior. Children were generally between the ages of 6 and 12 years, though some samples included older adolescents:

The diagnosis neurotic was made in those cases in which the manifestations of, or defenses against, anxiety were predominant . . . some of these children might have been classified under the rubric: adjustment reaction of childhood, neurotic traits. . . . Children who were overactive, distractible, non-conforming and disturbing to others, but who showed little or no anxiety, were classified as hyperkinetic . . . children with sociopathic behavior were *not* included in this category. (Eisenberg et al., 1961, p. 1088)

Because a symptom list on each child was completed by the parents at the time of diagnosis, it is possible to get some idea of which complaints first brought the children to the clinic. Each symptom was presented under one of 24 different problem areas familiar to parents, such as problems sleeping and problems with friends. For example, the problem headed "restlessness" included items of "restless or overactive," "excitable, impulsive," and "fails to finish things he starts (short attention span)." (The symptom list, somewhat modified by us in later revisions, is reproduced in Appendix A.)

We compared 360 of these children with 378 children matched for age, sex, race, and social class (Conners, 1970). Figure 2.1 presents these problem areas, ranked in the order in which they differ between the clinic and normal samples. As expected, almost all of the problem scores were significantly higher in the clinic sample, with school problems, restlessness, immaturity, and fears and worries being the most prominent in the clinic sample.

Within the clinic sample, a similar comparison can be made between the neurotic and hyperkinetic diagnoses (Figure 2.2), where it may be seen that problems of restlessness and keeping friends most characterize the hyperkinetics, while fears and worries and psychosomatic complaints characterize the neurotics.

However, the significant differences do not describe how these parent-defined problems *independently* contribute to the diagnosis. By using a discriminant function analysis we can calculate the weight that maximally discriminates the two diagnostic groups for each problem area. When this is done (Figure 2.3) it is plain that the *problem of restlessness is much more important* as a discriminator of the two groups compared with the next most important group of problems (keeping friends; fears and worries).

These results at a symptomatic level tend to validate the global diagnosis, which is hardly surprising since it is parents who bring their children to the clinic in the first place and describe the complaints that form part of the basis for the diagnosis. It would be an embarrassment if diagnosis were so haphazard that the hyperkinetics were found to be no less restless or more anxious than the neurotics!

SYMPTOMS IN CLINIC VS. CONTROL PATIENT

STUDENT'S T-TEST

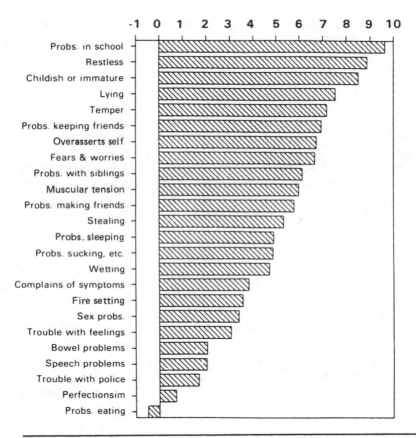

Figure 2.1. Parent ratings on 24 symptom categories for clinic patients (N = 360) versus matched controls (N = 378). Controls were matched with patients on sex, age, and social class. A t-test of approximately 2.0 is significant at the 5% level.

Response to Treatment

For a diagnosis to be meaningful, it must do more than provide an adequate symptomatic description. It must have some predictive validity regarding such important clinical issues as response to treatment

HYPERKINETIC VS. NEUROTIC
SYMPTOM DIFFERENCES

STUDENT'S T-TEST

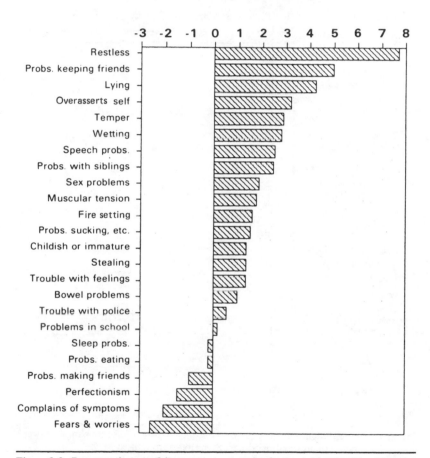

Figure 2.2. Parent ratings on 24 symptom categories for hyperkinetics (N = 120) and neurotics (N = 133).

(Klein, Gittelman, Quitkin, & Rifkin, 1980). The treatment studies described above had explored a number of drugs, including various sedatives and tranquilizers, as well as brief psychotherapy and counsel-

HYPERKINETIC VS. NEUROTIC
SYMPTOM DIFFERENCES

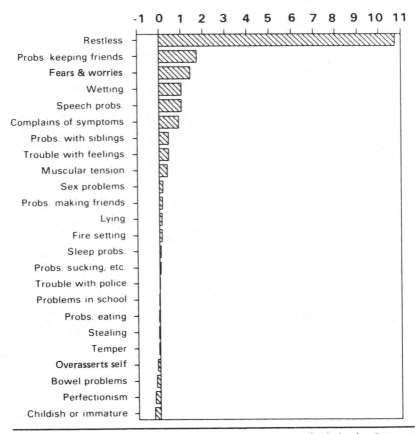

DISCRIMINANT FUNCTION SCORE
(THOUSANDS)

Figure 2.3. Independent contribution of symptom scores to discrimination between hyperkinetics and neurotics. Symptoms are ranked in the order of their independent contribution to the discrimination between neurotics and hyperkinetics.

ing. Using global clinical criteria of improvement, none of these treatments was found to be more effective than any other, so that by collapsing across types of treatment one can observe the effects of diagnosis upon outcome (Figure 2.4). Whereas almost 70% of the neurotics are

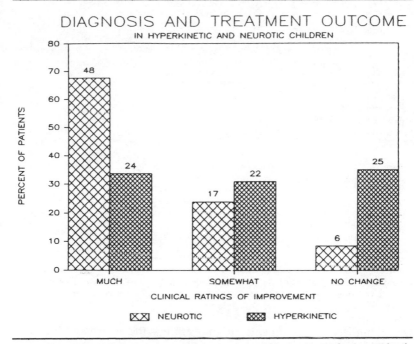

Figure 2.4. Global clinical ratings of improvement with treatment for hyperkinetic and neurotic patients. Data are collapsed across a variety of treatments that included brief psychotherapy, placebo, and various tranquilizing medications. None of the treatments was significantly different from any other, but differences between diagnoses are highly significant.

much improved over the 8 to 12 weeks of these studies, only about one-third of the hyperkinetics improve to a clinically significant degree. The reverse is true for the no-change category. Thus, diagnosis is a powerful predictor of treatment outcome (though at this point no *effective* treatments had been found). Having diagnosed these groups on clinical symptomatic grounds it is now possible to examine how they might differ in other respects, perhaps further validating the clinical diagnosis as well as giving us some insight into underlying mechanisms which distinguish hyperkinetic and neurotic children; or as we earlier referred to them, externalizing and internalizing children.

Intellectual Functioning

Fifty of the neurotics and 69 of the hyperkinetics had received the Wechsler Intelligence Scale for Children (WISC). The WISC Verbal IQ

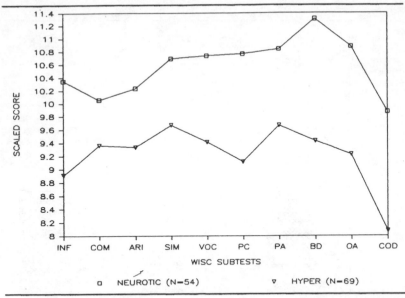

Figure 2.5. WISC profiles of neurotic and hyperkinetic patients illustrating the slight
intellectual disadvantage for hyperkinetics, especially for perceptual-
motor tasks.

was found to be significantly higher among the neurotics than the
hyperkinetics (about 6 points); but the Performance IQ was even more
significant (about 10 points). These results are in accord with many
studies that show a slight intellectual disadvantage for hyperkinetic and
learning disabled children (for a review, see E. D. Rie, in Rie & Rie,
1980).

A more informative picture emerges from the *pattern* of subtest
differences, as shown in Figure 2.5. The most significant difference is for
the picture completion task, followed by block design, coding, object
assembly, and picture arrangement. The two groups also differ on the
information and vocabulary subtests, but to a lesser degree. It seems
clear that the visual-perceptual-motor tasks are more difficult for the
hyperkinetics than the neurotics.

While it is not wise to make too much of these differences (Kaufman,
1979), as clinicians we may use these post hoc findings to develop
hypotheses, using what is known regarding the processes involved in the
different subtests. For example, there is evidence that relative deficits in
Performance IQ are associated with dysfunction in the right cerebral
hemisphere: Right-sided epileptic foci in children and other right-
hemisphere deficits are associated with lower Performance than Verbal
IQ (Fedio & Mirsky, 1969; Kershner & King, 1974; Rourke & Telegdy,
1971; Rudel & Teuber, 1971; Rudel, Teuber, & Twitchell, 1974).

Planning and Forethought

Another cognitive test of particular interest is the Porteus Mazes. The test requires that the subject find his way out of a pencil-maze, trying not to go into blind alleys or touch the sides of the maze. Because the child has as much time as needed to plan his way out, the Porteus IQ score is thought to primarily reflect planning and forethought. The Qualitative or Q-score more specifically reflects the child's attention to "the rules of the game," with high scores indicating motor impulsiveness (crossing the lines, touching sides of the maze), as well as failure to follow directions ("don't lift the pencil from the page"). Originally designed by Porteus to measure the intelligence of aboriginals (who performed well on maze-tracking but poorly on the Stanford-Binet), the Porteus IQ was the only measure from a large cognitive battery to show a decline in patients following frontal lobotomies in the Columbia-Greystone project (Porteus, 1959).

Table 2.1 presents data comparing hyperkinetics and neurotics on the Porteus Mazes as well as several other measures. The neurotics are clearly superior on the Porteus IQ (a difference, however, that disappears when the hyperkinetics are treated with stimulant drugs). Similar findings with many other tests implies that the deficits are not due to limitations of capacity, but in the *use* of the child's available resources, a point to be further developed in our chapter on drug studies.

Mood

Clyde (1963) has developed a mood scale originally intended for adult psychopharmacology studies. We were interested to see how the parents would characterize the mood of their children before and after treatment. Parents used a Q-sort method to describe their children, and factor scores were computed using the factor structure described by Clyde based upon studies with adults.

The Friendly factor includes items such as feels good-natured, pleasant, kind, and warmhearted. The Aggression factor includes boastful, forceful, rude, and sarcastic behaviors. The Clearthinking factor includes items like efficient, alert, clearthinking, and able to concentrate. The Sleepy factor includes sleepy, drowsy, fatigued, and tired. The Unhappy factor includes sad, downhearted, troubled, and worried. Finally, the Dizzy factor includes items such as feeling sick to the stomach, dizzy, jittery, and shaky.

TABLE 2.1
Comparison of Clinically Diagnosed Neurotics and Hyperkinetics

	Neurotics		Hyperkinetics		
	M	SD	M	SD	t-Test
Cycle Mood Scale	(N = 42)		(N = 40)		
Friendly	50.5	11.1	54.6	9.3	−1.78
Aggressive	60.5	13.8	60.2	2.75	0.10
Clear-thinking	49.5	8.0	39.7	8.10	5.11***
Sleepy	46.4	9.6	45.1	7.5	0.65
Unhappy	47.3	6.1	43.7	6.0	2.63*
Dizzy	49.0	6.8	49.6	6.7	−0.42
Porteus Maze Quotient	118.0	16.3	103.3	17.4	3.91***
Manifest Anxiety Scale	(N = 50)		(N = 59)		
Anxiety score	21.8	8.9	20.4	8.0	0.87
Lie scale	2.8	2.5	4.1	2.8	−2.71**
Childrearing Attitudes	(N = 42)		(N = 40)		
Discipline	1.7	0.9	2.0	1.0	−1.60
Uncertainty	0.7	0.9	1.0	1.1	−1.27
Rejection	1.8	1.1	2.1	1.2	−1.26
Responsibility	1.7	0.7	1.5	0.8	1.45
Maternal Hostility (IPAT)	(N = 41)		(N = 38)		
Overt	17.0	7.6	16.5	6.9	0.31
Covert	14.6	6.3	13.6	6.0	0.75
Cattell-Peterson Problems	(N = 42)		(N = 41)		
Behavioral problems (psychiatrist)	13.9	6.8	25.3	6.8	−7.65***
Personality problems (psychiatrist)	20.8	6.5	13.1	5.8	5.73***
Behavioral problems (social worker)	17.1	9.9	25.1	8.9	−3.87***
Personality problems (social worker)	15.9	5.8	11.9	6.1	3.07**
Luria Tremograph Task	(N = 23)		(N = 21)		
Omissions	6.0		10.0		−2.48*
Commissions	12.7		14.6		−2.54*
Multiple responses	2.8		5.2		−2.10*
Involuntary (nondominant response)	13.7		17.4		−2.19

*p < .05; **p < .01; ***p < .001 (two-tailed test).

The results indicate that parents of hyperkinetics describe their children as much less clearthinking and less unhappy than do mothers of neurotic children. It is important that mothers of hyperkinetics do *not* see their children as being more aggressive, but in fact see them as somewhat higher in friendliness than mothers of neurotics see their children. (Of course, only the child can directly access his own internal mood state, so these opinions of mothers are best regarded as statements by the parents of how they *perceive* their children's behavior rather than measures of the actual behaviors of the children.)

Maternal Attitudes and Personality

It might be supposed that if hyperkinetics are just poorly managed, undisciplined problem children, their mothers might favor either overly stringent or lax discipline, display more uncertainty regarding child management, engage in more rejection of the child, or be unwilling to take appropriate responsibility for the child's misconduct.

These attitude dimensions were identified from factor analysis by Gildea, Glidewell, and Kantor (1961), and were given to the parents of neurotic and hyperkinetic children in a 17-item questionnaire. Items for the Discipline factor include such statements as "Parents who are strict ought to know ahead of time what their children will and will not do." The Responsibility factor includes items like "Problems in children come out of troubles inside the family." Rejection is indicated by statements like "Jealousy is just a sign of selfishness in children." Uncertainty includes items such as "It's hard to know what healthy sex ideas are." No differences between neurotics and hyperkinetics in these general parenting attitudes were found.

A measure of maternal overt and covert anxiety also showed no differences between groups, using a self-report form by Cattell (1957). Because this measure also relies upon parental self-report, one may question its validity as a true measure of parental anxiety. But insofar as the test reflects conscious awareness and willingness to disclose subjective anxiety, it suggests that mothers of hyperkinetics are not more neurotically anxious than other clinic mothers.

Clinician Symptom Ratings

Table 2.2 presents a list of the 55 most common behavior and personality problems found in middle childhood (Peterson, 1961). In our studies the diagnosing psychiatrist and social worker were independently asked to check off these symptoms as present or absent. Both sources agree in finding significantly more behavior problems in the hyperkinetics, and significantly more personality problems in the neurotics. The correlation between psychiatrist and social worker ratings was significantly higher for behavior problems ($r = .61$) than for personality problems ($r = .17$), indicating that externalizing symptoms are more reliably recognized than personality problems.

TABLE 2.2
The 55 Most Common Symptoms of Middle Childhood

Conduct Problem	Personality Problem
Disobedience	Feelings of inferiority
Disruptiveness	Lack of self-confidence
Boisterousness	Social withdrawal
Fighting	Proneness to frustration
Attention-seeking	Self-consciousness
Restlessness	Shyness
Negativism	Anxiety
Impertinence	Lethargy
Destructiveness	Inability to have fun
Irritability	Depression
Temper tantrums	Reticence
Hyperactivity	Hypersensitivity
Profanity	Drowsiness
Jealousy	Aloofness
Uncooperativeness	Preoccupation
Distractibility	Lack of interest in environment
Irresponsibility	Clumsiness
Inattentiveness	Daydreaming
Laziness in school	Tension
Shortness of attention span	Suggestibility
Dislike for school	Crying
Nervousness	Preference for younger playmates
Thumbsucking	Specific fears
Skin allergy	Stuttering
	Headaches
	Nausea
	Truancy from school
	Stomachaches
	Preference for older playmates
	Masturbation
	Hay fever or asthma

SOURCE: From Peterson (1961). Reprinted with permission of the author.

Motor Inhibition

Alexander Luria (1960) was one of the first psychologists to demonstrate how motor behavior could be used to measure degree of voluntary control processes. He used a simple tremorgraph that recorded a subject's voluntary and involuntary motor responses in the face of disruptive emotional states. After the Russian revolution there were hundreds of people lined up for examinations that essentially would send them to the university or to Siberia. Luria recorded their motor responses to simple verbal commands before and after the examinations. He found that emotional states could significantly disrupt motor control. Similarly, he showed how motor performance was disrupted by anxiety and guilt by studying criminals before and after confession. In later studies (Luria & Yudovichy, 1959) he showed how the development of control over motor behavior in children was linked to their development of verbal self-regulation.

We utilized this method in studying the ability of hyperkinetic and neurotic children to inhibit and control motor behavior. A subject rested his hands on a platform connected to a flexible pneumatic bellows which recorded small hand movements on an ink-writing polygraph (Figure 2.6).

In our first study, children heard a series of words at 10-second intervals with the occasional word "press" interspersed. Upon hearing the word press they were supposed to press the right hand, but keep the left hand still. Responses to the wrong word were counted as commissions, and failure to respond as omissions. Responses of the nondominant hand were counted as involuntary responses. As shown in Table 2.1, the hyperkinetic subjects made significantly more omissions and commissions, but not more involuntary responses. They also made more multiple responses with the dominant hand. These findings suggested the hypothesis that hyperkinetics and neurotics differ in their ability to *voluntarily* inhibit motor response.

Habituation and Motor Control

Habituation is one of the most fundamental of all adaptive processes. Throughout all animal species a repeated stimulus results in a decrement in the magnitude of the original response when the stimulus has no appetitive consequences for the organism. At the same time, the subject can be required to give a voluntary motor response.

One way to tackle this problem is to disrupt motor control by a powerful stimulus, repeating the same stimulus a number of times and seeing how rapidly its disruptive effects diminish with repetition. When sudden, loud stimuli first occur, they evoke a massive startle response, which includes flexion of the arms, arching of the torso, widening of the mouth, and eyeblink (Landis & Hunt, 1939). This response pattern is a reflex response controlled by subcortical mechanisms. However, as the

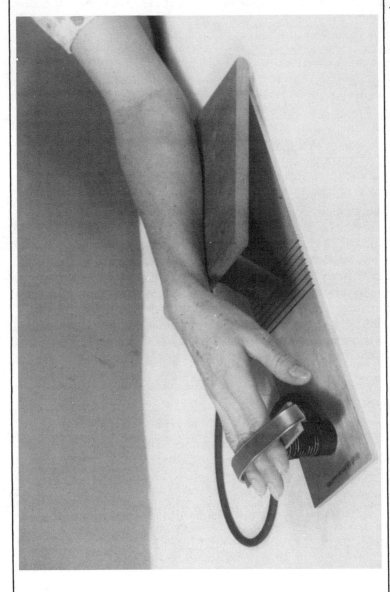

Figure 2.6. Tremorgraph for measuring motor control. Both hands rest on the pneumatic bellows, which is connected to a polygraph. Both voluntary and involuntary motor responses are recorded.

startle stimulus is repeated, higher cortical mechanisms come into play, and components of the startle response habituate[1] (Davis, 1948).

We carried out an experiment to determine whether the greater motoric response of hyperkinetics in the Luria tremorgraph was due to a deficiency in higher cortical inhibitory functions, or to deficiencies at a subcortical level (Conners & Greenfeld, 1966). Fifteen hyperkinetics (mean age = 10.0) were matched with 14 neurotics (mean age = 10.1). The children were told they would hear some very loud noises, which would make them jump, and that each time they heard the noise they should make a press with the right (dominant) hand, and leave the left hand absolutely still. A starter's pistol was fired out of sight, producing a very loud sound. This was repeated 12 times. The amplitudes of the voluntary and involuntary responses were measured. Both the left and right hands habituated, but the hyperkinetics were significantly slower in habituating with the *voluntary* hand. They did not differ from neurotics in habituation of the involuntary hand (Figure 2.7). We took these results to mean that hyperkinetics have a defect in higher cortical inhibitory mechanisms related to voluntary control over motor behavior, not simply deficits in habituation at the spinal level of control.

Younger children also habituated more slowly than older children, but the age effects were limited to the *involuntary* motor control responses. The involuntary movements (which have figured so prominently in theories related to neurological dysfunction) were characteristic of younger children, but not different between neurotic and hyperkinetic children. This finding suggests that immaturity over involuntary motor control may reflect maturational processes in the motor system which are independent of the defects in voluntary motor inhibition.

Perceptual Style

Despite the vivid clinical descriptions of hyperkinetic children, surprisingly little has been said about them from the point of view of classical clinical psychological techniques. During the time we were able to observe the psychiatrically defined hyperkinetic and neurotic samples, we decided to investigate their response to the inkblot test.

Notorious and controversial for its unreliability and dependence upon subjective clinical interpretation, the standard Rorschach test is not well suited to research investigations. However, a major advance in the use of this technique was provided by Holtzman (1961). In his version of the test, the subject is asked to give only one response to each

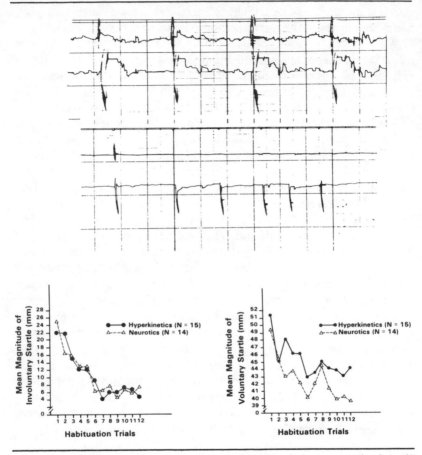

Figure 2.7. (a) Sample tremorgraph responses of patients in response to loud startle stimulus. Children are required to keep the left hand still and make a depression with the right hand on hearing the extremely startling noise. The first two tracings are from a very reactive child. Upper tracing is left hand; lower is right hand. Bottom tracings are from a well-controlled neurotic child. Note how this child immediately learns to control the left hand and gives smooth response with the right hand. (b) Habituation responses of left and right hands to 12 repeated startle stimuli for neurotics and hyperkinetics. Neurotics habituate more rapidly when voluntary control is required but not for involuntary (left-hand) responses. Other data (not shown) indicate that involuntary motor control shows a strong age-related development. From Conners and Greenfeld (1966, pp. 127-128). Reprinted with permission of publisher.

of 45 stimulus cards. Each card has been designed to pull for different response characteristics. Scoring is objective and reliable and covers 22 separate response categories, some derived from the Rorschach, but others (such as Barrier and Penetration) related to more recent work.

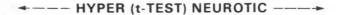

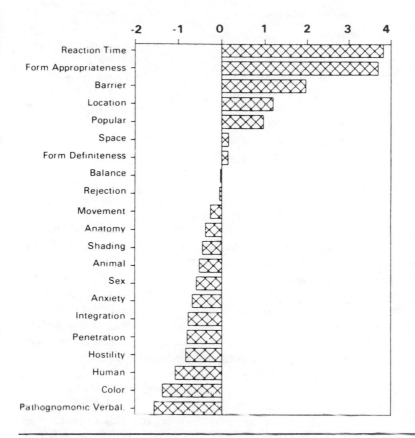

Figure 2.8. t-test of differences on 22 response categories from Holtzman Inkblot Test. Neurotics have longer reaction times, more form-appropriate and "bounded" responses; hyperkinetics show more color and deviant verbalizations. A t of 1.96 is significant at the 5% level (two-tailed test).

The 22 variables have been factor analyzed, revealing five independent and stable factors. Extensive validation studies and normative data for children and adults has been summarized by Hill (1972).

We administered the Holtzman Inkblot Technique (HIT) to 36 neurotic and 35 hyperkinetic children. The protocols were scored blindly by Holtzman's trained scorers. The results are presented in Figure 2.8. The hyperkinetics show significantly faster response times and lower form-appropriateness to the blots. They also have lower scores on the Perceptual Differentiation factor and Inhibition factor. Table 2.3 presents the composition and interpretation of the five HIT factors.

TABLE 2.3

Composition and Interpretation of Holtzman Inkblot Factors

Factor	Variables Included	Interpretation
I	Integration, movement, human, popular, form-definiteness, barrier, penetration (reversed)	Perceptual maturity and integrated ideational activity
II	Color, shading, form-definiteness (reversed)	Perceptual sensitivity
III	Pathognomonic verbalization, anxiety, hostility, movement	Psychopathology of thought
IV	Location, form-appropriateness	Perceptual differentiation
V	Reaction time, rejection animal (reversed)	Inhibition versus impulsivity

Reaction time to the inkblots is more liberally interpreted than in laboratory reaction time studies as "an index of the complexity of the inner process for a specific response" and the ability "to consciously direct thinking, concentrate on a task, and demonstrate the availability of inner resources" (Hill, 1972, p. 39). Form appropriateness (FA), the ability to verbalize a percept that is appropriate to the blot, is said to reflect several processes. First, it reflects "a conscious effort of attention to the distinctive features of the stimulus as separate from the needs of the viewer" (Hill, p. 50). FA also reflects ego control and the ability to control emotional impulsivity.

Lapses in attention due to an unbridled temper and lack of ability to concentrate have been described for people with low FA (Hill, 1972, p. 50). Derived as they are from a very different tradition of psychological investigation, these hypotheses from the inkblot performance of hyperkinetics are surprisingly concordant with our hypothesis regarding voluntary control processes in hyperkinetics. Each of the differences of hyperkinetics and neurotics on the HIT relate to *conscious efforts of control over impulse and the direction of attention.*

One additional finding was that the hyperkinetic children as a group are significantly more *variable* in reaction time, as well as more impulsive. Increased intrasubject variability in reaction time is typical of hyperkinetics (Cohen & Douglas, 1972; Sroufe, Sonies, West, & Wright, 1973). The greater intrasubject variability in hyperkinetics extends to autonomic arousal levels, and as described later, to motoneuron excitability and motor activity during sleep. This variability in performance was one of the symptomatic hallmarks cited by Laufer and Denhoff, and has led some authors to propose that hyperkinesis is a disorder of modulation or control (Gorenstein & Newman, 1980; Zentall & Zentall, 1983; Douglas & Peters, 1979; Hicks & Gualtieri, unpublished).

Low scores on Factor IV, Perceptual Differentiation, are said to reflect immaturity, diffuse body preoccupation with thought disturbances, and possible psychopathology (Holtzman, Thorpe, Swartz, and Herron, 1961). Factor V, Inhibition versus Impulsivity, "reflects the ability to respond to the total testing situation" (Hill, 1972, p. 141). On the whole, there appears to be a surprising concordance between the blind inkblot diagnosis and the classical description of the hyperkinetic child.

SYMPTOM DIMENSIONS AND TYPES

The clinicians in this study were clearly able to select patients who, in a broad sense, met the criteria for neurotic and hyperkinetic children; or as we prefer to think of them, as internalizing and externalizing. But most diagnosticians today would be distressed by the broad and global nature of this dichotomy, and would expect that important distinctions are being blurred by the global diagnosis. In particular, analysis of the behavior problem checklist indicates that a wide variety of conduct disturbances and aggressive behavior are being lumped together.

Factor analysis is a method of determining the minimum number of dimensions which can account for the correlations or shared variance among items. It is therefore of interest to see what factor dimensions describe the 93 items on the parent checklist. The factor matrix has been presented elsewhere (Conners, 1973). Table 2.4 presents the items that load most highly on each of the factors.

The results clearly show that conduct disorder and hyperactivity emerge as separate dimensions. This is in contrast to Quay (1979) and many others, who report either that items emerge as one factor or that the factors are highly correlated. Given that by definition factors are orthogonal, this has been a puzzle to Quay and others. This finding has been used as an argument that hyperactivity and conduct disorder are basically the same thing (Shaffer & Greenhill, 1979). The argument is also frequently made that hyperkinesis (or minimal brain dysfunction) cannot be a syndrome because the purported elements of the syndrome do not emerge on a common factor (Ross & Ross, 1982; Werry, 1968).

However, there are several reasons for discounting these arguments. First, factor-analytic studies which fail to find a hyperactivity factor usually restrict the number of factors, thus forcing them to load on a

TABLE 2.4
Factor Analysis of Parent Symptom Questionnaire

Factor/Item	Loading
Conduct Problem	
Bullying	.69
Bragging and boasting	.61
Sassy to grown-ups	.65
Mean	.71
Fights constantly	.67
Picks on other children	.69
Blames others for his mistakes	.67
Anxiety	
Afraid of new situations	.66
Afraid of people	.71
Afraid of being alone	.40
Worries about illness and death	.42
Shy	.57
Is afraid to go to school	.61
Afraid they do not like him	.50
Impulsive-Hyperactive	
Inattentive, easily distracted	NI*
Constantly fidgeting	NI
Cannot be left alone	.52
Always climbing	.55
A very early riser	.32
Will run around between mouthfuls at meals	.57
Unable to stop a repetitive activity	.56
Acts as if driven by a motor	.68
Learning Problem	
Is not learning	.60
Does not like school	.51
Will not obey school rules	.59
Has no friends	.47
Psychosomatic	
Awakens at night	.48
Headaches	.65
Stomach aches	.71
Vomiting	.56
Aches and pains	.65
Perfectionism	
Everything must be just so	.78
Things must be done same way every time	.72
Sets goals that are too high	.64
Antisocial	
Steals from parents	.54
Steals at school	.60
Steals from schools and other places	.68
Gets into trouble with police	.52

*NI = Item not included in original factor analysis.

single factor. Second, the size and breadth of the item pool will determine whether few or many factors emerge (Lahey, Stempniak, Robinson, & Tyroler, 1978). Third, it should be recalled that factor analysis provides independent *dimensions on which items load,* not *types of individuals.* Finally, the use of unit weights rather than factor score coefficients in computing factor scores will build in correlations between factors when scored on a new sample; it is the *independent* contribution of items that is needed. Thus, factor score coefficients rather than unit factor weights should be used to weight the items before summing. These scores weighted by factor coefficients are comparable to a linear combination of *independent* predictors in a multiple regression equation.

We reanalyzed our parent symptom data and found that the correlation between the Hyperactive-Immature factor and Conduct Disorder factor using unit weights on a new sample was .82 when applied to a new test sample. But this correlation dropped to .20 when the factor score coefficients were used instead of unit weights. This correlation, while still significant, represents only a 4% overlap in variance between the two factor dimensions in the replication sample (Blouin, Conners, & Seidel, unpublished).

In sum, we believe that restrictive item pools, small numbers of factors extracted, biased clinical samples, and statistical artifact account for the misguided belief that conduct disorders and hyperkinesis represent the same basic disorder. It is a different question, however, when one asks what *combinations* of these factors actually appear in clinical samples. A different method is required to identify which combinations of the underlying factor dimensions occur in clinical practice.

CLUSTER TYPES

What then are the natural groupings of children who appear at the outpatient clinic? Given that the *factors* discovered in the complaints of parents may represent orthogonal (independent) dimensions, do those dimensions intersect in ways that produce recognizable *types of individuals*? One possibility is that all possible types are represented. Thus, with eight independent symptom dimensions that could take on only two states (say above or below the median), there are 2^8 or 256 possible types. This is clearly too refined a categorization to be clinically meaningful! But it is an empirical question as to how many of the possible types actually occur in a clinic sample. (Presumably those that do not appear at the clinic either do not exist or, more likely, are not viewed as pathological by those parents who experience them, and so are not referred.)

A variety of computer algorithms can sort people into clusters based on the distance in N-dimensional space between their factor profiles. One can stop clustering when all or most individuals are classified. In effect, people whose profile of tests or symptoms are similar are lumped together. Different clustering algorithms produce somewhat different results, depending upon the type of data (Edelbrock & McLaughlin, 1980), and these methods are useless if one happens not to include the relevant dimensions needed to define the entity in question (see Klein et al., 1980, for a straightforward discussion of limitations of clustering in psychiatric diagnosis).

Using the factor dimensions of the parent questionnaire, we employed cluster analysis on 316 clinic patients and 365 normals from our sample. Using "the magic number seven, plus or minus two" as a reasonable number of cluster types to employ, we limited the number of clusters to five and obtained the profiles shown in Figure 2.9.

Cluster 1 appears to resemble an antisocial, learning-disabled conduct disorder. Cluster 2 clearly includes the classically neurotic child who is anxious, psychosomatic, and immature. Cluster 3 is a group high on the restless-impulsive dimension, moderately immature and moderately high on conduct disorder. Cluster 4 is entirely defined by the small group of items representing perfectionistic tendencies ("things must be just so"; "sets too high goals"), and Cluster 5 are presumably normals (insofar as they have scores that are lower across the board, and a very flat profile).

It is also of interest that the hyperkinetic cluster (Cluster 3) has a moderate elevation on conduct disturbance. Our arguments above notwithstanding, it seems that there is some overlap *in this clinic sample* between conduct disturbances and restless impulsivity. One hypothesis that accounts for this fact is that conduct disorder itself is a heterogeneous cluster of symptoms, with some individuals experiencing secondary symptoms to their hyperkinesis, while others have some form of primary aggressive-spectrum disorder. Evidence for the secondary nature of aggressive symptomatology will be discussed in Chapter 7. Sampling problems with clinically referred children would tend to preclude the identification of separate aggressive and hyperactive types, assuming that it is more likely that children with both disorders get referred most often.

The work of Trites and Laprade (1983) supports the conclusion that the two dimensions are independent. They sampled teacher ratings on over 14,000 normal Canadian schoolchildren with our teacher ques-

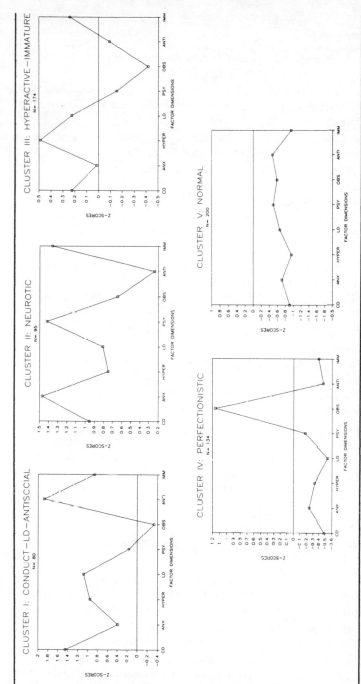

Figure 2.9. Symptom patterns derived from cluster analysis. The ordinate is in standard deviation units. CD = Conduct Disorder, Anx = Anxious, Hyper = Hyperactive/Impulsive, LD = Learning Disorder, Psy = Psychosomatic, Obs = Obsessional, Anti = Antisocial, Imm = Immature/Inattentive.

tionnaire and examined the independent clusters that are composed by the intersection of the factors arising from the questionnaire. Using a criterion of two standard deviations, about 1% of the children were exclusively hyperactive and nonconduct disordered or highly emotional. When the two traits of hyperactivity and conduct disorder are confounded, there are about 3.7% who are high on both. These prevalence figures approximate those reported by English investigators who tend to restrict the term hyperkinesis to relatively severe cases (Sandberg, Rutter, & Taylor, 1978).

If these naturally occurring types in the clinic represent reasonably distinct entities, how do they relate to the clinical diagnoses based upon a more global differentiation into hyperkinetic and neurotic? Figure 2.10 shows the percentage of diagnosed neurotics and hyperkinetics who appear in each of the empirically derived cluster domains. As we might hope, Cluster 3 (restless/impulsive and inattentive/immature) does contain the largest number of diagnosed hyperkinetics, but just barely. Almost 70% of the clinically diagnosed hyperkinetics are distributed among the other types, with many of them assigned to the group high on antisocial and aggressive conduct. This means, at least with respect to the empirically defined clusters, that the clinicians have included quite heterogeneous groups within their broad diagnosis of hyperkinesis.

Some diagnosed hyperkinetics will plainly be quite anxious and aggressive while others will not. Conversely many children diagnosed by clinicians as neurotic should perhaps have found their proper home in Cluster 3 along with their hyperkinetic peers. The simple dichotomy employed in these early drug studies is clearly insufficient to account for the variety of symptom patterns which actually occur, at least as the symptoms are defined by parental report.

SUMMARY AND DISCUSSION

The studies reported here are based on a broad, somewhat loose and global clinical diagnosis, but a diagnosis made by experienced child psychiatrists with access to comprehensive clinical and background data. The diagnosis reflects an integrative synthesis of information derived from parents, teachers, examinations, interviews, and historical data. Despite the obvious weaknesses in this procedure, it probably represents a good standard of clinical practice. The type of differences between diagnoses on a number of variables argues for the validity of the

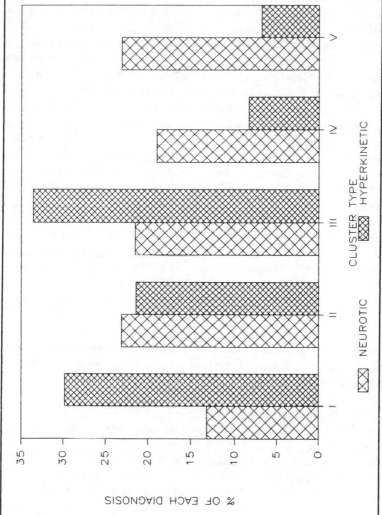

Figure 2.10. Percentage of clinically diagnosed neurotics and hyperkinetics who fall into types defined by cluster analysis. Identification of cluster types as in Figure 2.9.

conceptual distinction between these disorders as internalizing and externalizing.

Our studies of this sample show that restlessness is the single most discriminating symptom between neurotic and hyperkinetic children. But the clinicians also attribute more behavior problems of all kinds to hyperkinetics than to comparable neurotic children. This validation procedure is reassuring but, because of its circular nature, only weakly compelling. The fact that hyperkinetics are markedly less responsive to treatments of all kinds, including psychotherapy, counseling, sedatives, and tranquilizing drugs, is a much more compelling argument that there are fundamental differences among the diagnostic groups.

Intellectually, although within the normal range, the hyperkinetics show lower performance on tests presumably tapping right hemisphere function. Their vocabulary and stored information are also lower, consistent with the high incidence of school related symptomatology; but other measures of intellectual ability such as general comprehension and abstract thinking are not different from neurotics, as are parent judgments of efficiency, alertness, and concentration. Thus, it is not just that hyperactives are less intellectually competent, but they have a particular form of intellective dysfunction centering on poor planning and forethought and visual-constructional-spatial tasks.

While our information about the parents themselves is limited to self-reports, maternal anxiety and dimensions of parental attitudes are not different between neurotics and hyperkinetics, leading us to conclude at this point that parental attitudes play a relatively minor role in the genesis of hyperkinesis. (Such findings of course, say nothing regarding actual parental *behavior*—an issue to be dealt with later.)

Voluntary motor inhibition is distinctly poorer for hyperkinetic children, but not automatic motor processes linked to maturation. They show a lack of ability to gain control over voluntary motor behavior in the face of strong, disinhibiting stimuli but regain motor control at the same rate as neurotics, suggesting that their deficits are at a higher cortical level where the *intentionality* of the motor act is involved. It seems quite possible however, that involuntary motor deficits can intersect with many other disorders; maturationally related motor phenomena will be discussed in more detail in our chapter on motor behavior.

The externalizing children's response to ambiguous perceptual stimuli is characterized by impulsiveness and lack of differentiation of the stimuli into discrete structures. They may be said to have an impulsive perceptual style as well as an impulsive motoric style.

The data strongly suggest that there are independent dimensions of symptomatic behavior, that they are patterned in recognizable ways, that only a limited subset of the possible combinations appears in the clinic, and that clinician DSM-II diagnoses are too broad to encompass the variety of complaints that parents make about their children. The broad band categories of hyperkinesis and neurosis certainly have some validity in terms of treatment responsiveness, cognitive and perceptual styles, and disinhibitory behavior. Only when we wish to narrow our focus and make finer distinctions do we find other symptom dimensions to be intermixed within the original dichotomous groups.

It is our opinion that much of the polemic in the literature regarding the existence of a syndrome is simply a disagreement about the level of analysis and the type of operations employed in arriving at a classification scheme. Do broad categories exist which conform with the Laufer and Denhoff syndrome, and which clinicians can reliably recognize? Apparently the answer is yes; our clinical study confirms that the psychiatric diagnoses are associated with a number of objective differences that are consistent with the basic syndrome described by Laufer and Denhoff.

But are these broad dimensions *too* broad according to more objective symptomatic criteria? Our data appear to suggest the affirmative. Psychiatrists using DSM-II appear to have assigned patients on the basis of only two of several different symptom dimensions, thus blurring distinctions among separate types that can be recognized by empirical clustering methods. Nevertheless, the concept of a hyperkinetic behavior syndrome has served a useful function as the basis for a bootstrapping operation in which measures associated with the syndrome have been identified, and which can then be used to refine classification. In subsequent chapters we will examine the implications of a still more differentiated view of these children, going beyond the surface phenomena of observable symptoms as recorded by parents, teachers, and clinicians.

NOTE

1. It is thought that the subject's evaluation of the stimulus as being inconsequential or irrelevant influences the rate of habituation (O'Gorman, 1977). Soviet workers have tended to view habituation processes as reflective of the speed of generation of central, inhibitory processes (Nebylitsyn, 1972). Sokolov (1969) proposed that habituation is a function of cortical inhibitory control over subcortical arousal. Crider and Lunn (1971) demonstrated that habituation in the *vasomotor* system is an individual difference variable strongly related to extraverted, impulsive behavior. Subjects who habituate rapidly are more resistant to distraction (Siddle & Mangan, 1971). The ability to habituate to irrelevant task stimuli influences the degree to which those stimuli interfere with selective attention (Waters, McDonald, & Koresko, 1977).

3

THE NEUROPSYCHOLOGY OF HYPERACTIVITY

So far we have considered hyperkinesis primarily from a clinical, symptomatic point of view. Descriptions of the syndrome have usually been limited to grossly observable symptoms; more properly, complaints of others. The exception is the early observation of "visual perceptual" dysfunctions and academic functioning which were noticed from the outset by Laufer and Denhoff and repeatedly commented upon by others subsequently. While valuable, and indeed essential, complaints of behavior may tell us as much about the observers as about the child.

Disturbances of the central nervous system are more clearly reflected by probes of the child's performances on verbal, visual-spatial, and attentional tasks that underlie the child's negotiations with the physical and social environment. There are also certain functions that defy purely symptomatic characterization, such as planfulness, organization, and strategy. They reflect higher integrative cortical processes that are often too subtle to recognize within the flux of behavior because they are easily confused with other factors such as oppositional, aggressive, distractible, or motivational problems. For these reasons, we turn to a neuropsychological approach.

THE NEUROPSYCHOLOGICAL APPROACH

Neuropsychology is not defined by particular tests or measuring instruments, but by a way of looking at behavior. Neuropsychological reasoning does not depend upon a particular set of facts but rather upon patterns of facts organized by their presumed relationship to the structure and function of the brain. Speculations regarding brain-behavior relationships are hazardous because so much is unknown about the brain, and what is known shows an extraordinarily complex picture. Nevertheless, neuroanatomic and neurophysiological models provide useful hypotheses regarding the meaning of behavioral data. It is not *necessary* to invoke neural explanations of behavior but it is sometimes helpful in understanding why certain behaviors are organized in a particular way.

Good examples of this approach are the attempts to establish parallels between septal defects and disinhibitory psychopathology (Gorenstein & Newman, 1980), and between anxiety and septo-hippocampal defects (Gray, 1982). Gray's theory has been extended to attempt to account for the syndrome of minimal brain dysfunction (Bloomingdale, Davies, & Gold, 1984). Quay (in press) has used this model to generate differential predictions regarding reward and avoidance learning and to account for inconsistencies in autonomic function among hyperkinetic children.

However, certain principles of brain function have a chastening influence upon neuropsychological speculation. First, everything is connected to everything else. Hardly any part of the brain can be understood as the single locus from which some behavioral function emerges *de novo*. Since the time of Sherrington, it has been conventional to regard brain functions as being interlocked in an orderly, hierarchical cybernetic chain of influences (Brobeck, 1979). Such an arrangement helps us understand how apparently quite different behaviors such as paying attention, aggressive behavior, and restlessness may be localized in specific parts of the brain, while at the same time depending upon common resources in several widely dispersed brain regions.

Second, there is considerable redundancy in the brain. Many functions are represented or rerepresented among quite different structures, making it difficult to know which brain sites influence which behavioral events. A particular defect in activity level or attention or language may result from any number of lesions or from interactions among different parts of the nervous system. Especially among children, we know that recovery from damage depends upon the inherent plasticity of the brain and its ability to reorganize itself to accommodate the damage (Rourke, Bakker, Fisk, & Strang, 1983). Maturation of the brain and developmental progressions are characterized by increasingly greater interconnectivity among existing structures at the same time that entirely new structures and functional systems are emerging. This shifting topography of the brain in the face of development as well as insult confounds easy explanations of how current function relates to particular brain processes.

Nevertheless, we know that the adult brain does become highly specialized in particular ways with respect to functions of language, spatial analysis, planning and forethought, attention, and motor behavior. Undisturbed, the child's brain evolves toward recognizable specificity in the way various cognitive and behavioral functions are organized and mapped onto the brain's structures. A rich tradition of surgical, electrical stimulation, and clinical neurological investigations has provided an important base for neuropsychological theory. More recently brain imaging techniques have provided further direct evidence of the way behavioral functions are related to regional anatomic, biochemical, and vascular pathways in the brain.

Finally, there is the important principle that the brain evolves throughout its lifetime in concert with the physical and social environment. The higher the mammalian species, the more dependent the brain is upon its transactions with the environment to fulfill its destiny. The human brain, particularly in a developing child, craves optimal stimulus input (Hebb, 1955). A good argument can be made that the human organism is constantly in the process of creating behavioral adjustments that modulate sensory input (Zentall & Zentall, 1983). These adjustments require constant transactions with the physical and social environment, and in the case of dysfunctional biological resources it is these transactions that lead to the observable symptomatology. Damage to the nervous system resulting in some primary disorganization leads to atypical relations with the physical and social environment and the patterns of behavior which we recognize as symptoms (Birch, 1964). As far as brain-behavior relationships are concerned, neuropsychology is thus a two-way street. With some of these caveats in mind, let us consider some speculations regarding the origins of the hyperkinetic behavior pattern.

POSSIBLE NEURAL MECHANISMS IN HYPERKINESIS

The clinical findings of the previous chapter, in combination with the remarkable calming action of stimulant drugs, led us very early to the belief that at least two different dimensions of brain activity must account for the findings: an activation system and an inhibitory system:

> The decrease in impulsivity (as measured by the Porteus Maze) and in aggressive behavior (as measured by symptom ratings) . . . is compatible with the hypothesis that methylphenidate enhances the action of inhibitory controlling systems. . . . However, a second mechanism—increased alerting— is probably active here if we are to judge from reports of human performance on stimulants and from the remarkably alert attitudes of primates whose spontaneous pacing has been decreased by these agents as opposed to tranquilizers. (Conners & Eisenberg, 1963, p. 462)

There are several possible brain mechanisms which might underlie the behavioral patterns of disinhibition and inattentiveness, and account for the effects of stimulants in altering these patterns.

Frontal Lobe Function

Although no adequate theory yet encompasses the functions of the large, cortical mass known as the frontal lobes (Jouandet & Gazzaniga, 1979), neuropsychological testing of subjects with known frontal lobe damage has provided a detailed picture of the cognitive and social behaviors mediated by the frontal lobes. The motor and premotor cortex involve both primary and secondary levels of motor control; that is, control over relatively discrete skilled movements, as well as more complexly integrated motor plans. The prefrontal areas provide a tertiary level of motor control, that is, the rerepresentation of plans for action and planning of sequences of behavior. In this way action patterns can be guided by "plans" that also serve as the basis for a continual update of progress in executing the plans. The heedlessness of hyperactive children is most suggestive of a failure in systems of maintaining and correcting action patterns.

As described in standard textbooks, damage to the frontal lobes produces a complex behavioral picture that is immediately of interest to students of hyperkinetic children:

(1) *Lack of restraint* leading to boasting, self-aggrandizement, hostility, and aggressiveness.
(2) *Distractibility* and *restlessness*, with difficulty in fixing attention.
(3) *Hypermotility,* which appears to be caused by the loss especially of area 13 on the orbital surface.

(4) *Flight of ideas*, puerile fantasies, emotional instability, facetiousness, and punning.

(5) *Lack of initiative* and difficulty in planning any course of action.

(6) *Impairment of memory* for recent events but not for remote events.

(7) *Impairment of moral and social sense,* loss of love for family.

(8) *Failure to realize*, or indifference to, the seriousness of his condition, and a sense of well-being (euphoria) (Brobeck, 1979, p. 125).

The similarity of frontal lobe dysfunctions and hyperkinetic impulse disorders has not escaped the attention of clinicians (Pontius, 1973), neurophysiologists (Stamm & Kreder, 1979), and neuropsychologists (Mattes, 1980; Hicks & Gualtieri, unpublished). The latter authors, reviewing evidence from animal models, symptom patterns, and neuropharmacology, find a close parallel between disturbances in frontal lobe functions and hyperkinetic behavior. According to them, similarities exist between the two syndromes in attention-distractibility, perseveration, minor motor abnormalities, impulse control, frustratibility, planning and judgment, socially disapproved behavior, emotional lability, and intrasubject variability.

One of the features of activity level in both humans and animals experiencing frontal lesions is that they are frequently *hypoactive* until stimulated. Davis (1957) described increased activity in frontally lesioned monkeys; the activity was recorded by a stabilimetric cage that tilted when the animals moved, and it was in fact the inability to *terminate* this impetus that accounted for their higher overall activity counts.[1] Thus, in the absence of frontal inhibition, there is a kind of behavioral inertia in response to stimulation. Novel or attractive stimuli may then exert undue influence over behavior, making it appear as though there is excessive distractibility, which is in fact diminished inhibition.

Brain Imaging in Hyperkinesis (ADD) and Learning Disorders

Recent techniques of brain imaging promise to reveal much more regarding the way higher intellectual functions are mapped onto the brain surface. For example, topographic electroencephalographic studies of dyslexic children reveal that the pattern of EEG activity is abnormal in several cortical regions traditionally believed to subserve reading and speech. However, there are differences between dyslexic and normal children that are not expected by classical aphasiology research in adults. The medial frontal lobe (supplementary motor area), the left lateral frontal lobe, the left midtemporal lobe, the left posterior quadrant (including Wernicke's area), and the left posterior parietal lobe, all show differences between normal and dyslexic groups (Duffy, Denckla, Bartels, & Sandini, 1980). Similar regions of activation have been found in cerebral blood flow studies during speech and during oral and silent reading (Larsen, Skinhoj, & Lassen, 1978; Lassen, Ingvar, & Skinhoj, 1978). These results therefore suggest that reading and verbal behavior constitute a complex functional system involving several discrete anatomical loci, and possibly different neurochemical systems as well. This system clearly overlaps with the functional systems proposed as underlying hyperkinesis, in both its attentional and inhibition aspects. The high degree of relationship between hyperkinetic behavior disorders and learning disorders may therefore derive from this intertwining of separate functional brain systems.

Spelling and verbal and design fluency are also affected by damage to the frontal lobes. Verbal expression, voluntary eye movements, perceptual differentiation, and recent memory are thought to rely, at least in part, upon frontal mechanisms. Expressive speech is subserved by Broca's area (left frontal cortex). These cognitive deficits are familiar, albeit inconsistent, accompaniments of the hyperkinetic syndrome.

In a recent application of another sophisticated brain imaging technique involving computer mapping of radio-isotope-labeled blood flow, more direct evidence has been provided for brain dysfunction in hyperkinetics. By examining the perfusion of the labeled dye into blood vessels it is possible to pinpoint areas of reduced function. Most impressively, all of the hyperactive children in these studies were found to have reduced perfusion of the labeled substance *bilaterally in the white matter of the frontal lobes,* and 7 of the 11 cases also had decreased perfusion in the caudate nuclei as well (Lou, Henriksen, & Bruhn, 1984).[2] Reduced blood flow in areas that included the basal ganglia and mesencephalon disappeared following methylphenidate treatment, suggesting that the drug was acting upon dopaminergic mechanisms in these areas, resulting in increased blood flow in central frontal regions regulating attention and impulse control. Another consequence of the drug treatment was a concomitant reduction of the perfusion in the motor cortex and primary sensory cortex, "suggesting an inhibition of function of these structures, seen clinically as less distractibility and decreased motor activity during treatment" (Lou et al., 1984, p. 829).

As yet, these brain imaging techniques have used small samples and have not provided corroborative neuropsychological behavioral measures, so they must be considered preliminary. But these results support the notion of an important role for frontal lobe regulatory mechanisms in hyperkinesis and related disorders.

The Reticular Activating System

This diffuse and ill-defined system of fibers occupies the central portion of the tegmentum of the brain stem. It is known to selectively facilitate or inhibit any movement. It projects fibers throughout the cortex, probably acting selectively to excite primary sensory areas and to inhibit other areas. It is presumed to be the modulator of stimulus arousal effects, acting to broaden or narrow attention in accordance with requirements for facilitating or gating out unwanted stimulation. This system has been described as the most critical integrative center of the brain, acting as a gating mechanism for all sensory influx, modulator of cortical function, readout mechanism for cortical differentiative and comparative processes, and gain manipulator for motor output (Scheibel & Scheibel, 1967).

Neurophysiologic evidence suggests that reticular nuclei of the thalamus subserve an inhibitory gating function for activity being relayed to the cortex (Skinner & Yingling, 1977; Yingling & Skinner, 1976). *The fact that these thalamic reticular nuclei are inhibited by activity in the mesencephalic reticular formation and selectively activated by the frontal cortex means that selective attention, arousal, and frontal lobe functions are linked together in an interdependent network.* As we shall see later, neurophysiological measures reveal an increase in certain types of frontal activity during the process of selective attending in hyperkinetics. Various lines of evidence support the hypothesis that these electrophysiologic changes reflect activity in the frontal-reticular loop (Picton, Campbell, Baribeau-Braun, & Prouix, 1978).

Maturation of the Frontal Lobes

Hyperkinesis is viewed by almost all observers as a developmental disorder. Some have specifically characterized it as a "maturational lag" disorder (Kinsbourne, 1973, 1979). It is of interest that myelination of neurons in the frontal lobes continues late into adolescence (Yakovlev & Lecours, 1967). Phylogenetically the most recent portion of the brain to mature, the lateral surfaces of the frontal cortex, in common with the inferior parietal area, are thought to develop last during ontogenesis (Nauta, 1971). These regions therefore hold the best potential for explanations of behavior based upon neurodevelopmental lag.

The Limbic System

In 1937 Papez proposed that a ring of structures comprising the older cortices surrounding the basal ganglia and contiguous with the neocortex were responsible for emotional and affective expression. MacLean (1949) reformulated the "Papez circuit" into the concept of the limbic system. Connections of this system with the hypothalamus are the means whereby both endocrine and autonomic effectors are controlled, thus giving it widespread influence throughout the body.

That there are many connections between the limbic system and the frontal lobe, particularly between limbic projections and the most anterior orbito-frontal areas known as Brodmann's areas 9, 10, 11, 12, 13, and 14 (Figure 3.1) is of considerable theoretical interest.

Subtle aspects of personality and social behavior appear to depend upon the orbital-frontal cortex and its interrelationships with the limbic-hypothalamic axis (Beaumont, 1983; Damasio & Hoesen, 1983). All indications are that the two systems are mutually regulatory, and in addition to the role of the frontal lobe in inhibiting fight-flight and emotional reactions, the limbic system is an important source of *afferent* input to the frontal cortex, increasing its inhibitory capacity.

In addition to influences upon orbito-frontal systems, on the basis of recent anatomical evidence it is highly likely that "many parts of the limbic system, and especially the limbic cortices, have rather wide-ranging inroads to key parts of the motor system" (Damasio & Hoesen, 1983, p. 92). Electrical stimulation of the cingulate portion of the limbic frontal lobe produces a "reaction of wakefulness" suggestive of heightened attention which arrests all other activity *except for* a variety of fidgety movements including impatient movements of the legs, suggestive of akathisia (Damasio & Hoesen, 1983, p. 101). This limbic area has been described as having a primary and general function of "inciting to action." These arrangements may clarify the reason for the excess of fidgeting activity which often takes place under conditions of high activation and attentional demand, such as when children are concentrating on schoolwork.

It was fortuitous in our earlier investigations that we studied hyperkinetic children who were deliberately contrasted with anxious neurotic

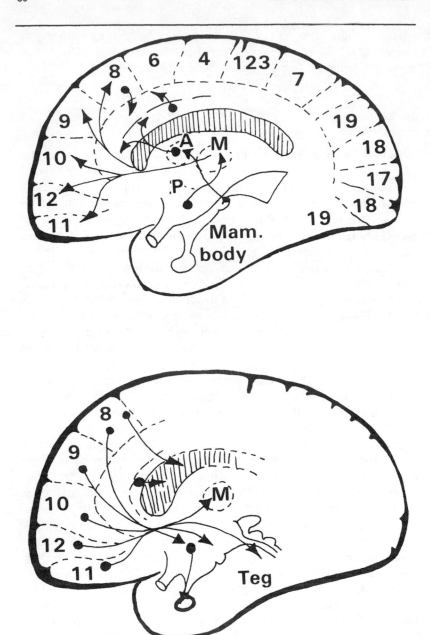

Figure 3.1. Mutual influence of frontal and limbic systems. (a) Cortical projections from limbic and thalamic areas to frontal cortex. (b) Frontal to limbic projections. After Brobeck (1979), Figure 9.118, © 1979 Williams and Wilkins, Baltimore. Reprinted with permission.

children. If the arousal, activation, and alerting responses associated with emotional stimuli are governed by limbic mechanisms (distinct from forebrain mechanisms involved in inhibition and control), those two patient groups should provide the sharpest possible contrast. (We will present evidence in the following chapter to show how anxiety levels affect resting and task arousal among hyperkinetics.)

It seems reasonable to assume that normal biological variation, as well as various forms of genetic influences or brain insult, can independently vary the dimensions of inhibition and activation/arousal through influences on frontal and thalamic/limbic systems, respectively. There would then be at least four main types of possible dysfunction, of which only two were being selected by our diagnostic practices: The impulsive and inattentive children would be those high on disinhibition and low on anxiety (hyperkinetics); the "neurotics" would be those with a combination of high inhibition and high anxiety. In addition, there should be types characterized by being disinhibited and anxious (neurotic impulse disorder?) and inhibited and nonanxious (hypoactive type?). The latter child, quite understandably, seldom finds his way into the clinic because he is a bother only to himself, not others.

NEUROPSYCHOLOGICAL PROFILES OF HYPERKINETIC CHILDREN

Over the course of several drug studies of hyperkinetic children, it was possible to obtain a variety of psychological measures tapping more specific functions than used in our earliest studies. In the later studies each child was screened for sensory defects, gross neurological status, and epilepsy by a pediatric neurologist. Family stability and psychopathology, situational stresses that might account for symptoms, psychosis, and overtly delinquent behavior resulting in arrests or judicial proceedings were assessed by a semistructured interview of the parents carried out by a child psychiatrist and social worker.

Children who were psychotic or delinquent, or whose families were disorganized, experiencing severe life stresses or parental psychopathology, were excluded from further study. A standardized psychiatric examination of the child (Rutter & Graham, 1968), in conjunction with the medical, social and developmental history, was used to exclude other primary psychiatric diagnoses. Only about 65% of children originally referred because of behavior or learning problems were included as meeting the criteria for hyperkinesis. The ages of the 262 children who remained in the protocols ranged from 61 to 156 months.

The sample was predominantly middle class, with the percentage of children falling in the five classes of the Hollingshead two-factor index of social position: 7.6, 22.3, 31.5, 25.9, and 12.7, for classes 1 to 5, respectively. Children had to have a Verbal or Performance IQ on the Wechsler Intelligence Scale for Children of 80 or above. They also had to score at least 1.5 standard deviations above the mean on either the parent or teacher hyperactivity factor from our teacher and parent rating scales.

The following measures were obtained on each child:

Wide Range Achievement Test (WRAT). This is an individually administered standardized achievement test measuring word recognition, spelling from dictation, and arithmetic. Scores are expressed in school grade levels (Jastak & Jastak, 1965).

Wechsler Intelligence Scale for Children (WISC). This is a standardized intelligence test that gives a full scale IQ, Verbal IQ, and Performance IQ (Wechsler, 1949).

Porteus Maze Test. This test consists of a series of progressively more difficult paper-and-pencil mazes to be solved (Porteus, 1965). The test is thought to be primarily a measure of planning, forethought, and impulsivity. The test quotient is comparable to an IQ score, with a normal mean of 100 and standard deviation of 15. The Q-score, or qualitative score, is a separate measure of how well the child follows directions regarding not touching the sides of the maze, lifting the pencil, and impulsivity. It has shown good validity in discriminating delinquents from other special populations.

Draw-A-Man Test. The child is asked to draw the best man he knows how to draw. The drawing is objectively scored for developmental level by the Harris-Goodenough scoring system (Harris, 1963). Results are expressed as a quotient with a mean of 100 and standard deviation of 15.

Bender-Gestalt Test. This test requires the child to copy ten progressively more complex geometric designs onto a single page. Accuracy of reproduction is scored by the Koppitz scoring method (Koppitz, 1964).

A higher score indicates more impairment of capacity to organize visual Gestalts.

Frostig Developmental Test of Visual Perception. This is a paper-and-pencil test that provides an overall perceptual quotient (PQ) and five subscores: eye-motor coordination, figure-ground, form constancy, position in space, and spatial relations. It also is standardized with a mean of 100 and standard deviation of 15 (Frostig, 1961). Because we have found the subscores to be highly intercorrelated, only the PQ is utilized here.

Paired-Associate Learning Test (PAL). This test consists of ten pairs of symbols and pictures that are repeated until the child correctly identifies all pairs or for a maximum of 16 trials through the list. Stimuli are presented automatically by a slide projector at 5-second intervals. Scores are number of trials to criterion and total number of errors. A high score indicates slower learning of the lists. Each trial through the list is presented in a different random order to minimize learning of serial position (Conners, Eisenberg, & Sharpe, 1964).

Continuous Performance Test (CPT). This test requires the child to monitor a panel of four displays that present stimuli made from orthogonal combinations of red-blue and horizontal-vertical lines in each of the four light displays. The child presses a fifth button in the center of the panel if one of the four target displays contains a red-vertical target. Three hundred trials are presented in which 50 contain the critical stimulus. A failure to respond to the critical stimulus within 1.6 seconds is counted as an error of omission. Responding when the critical stimulus is not presented is an error of commission. A higher score indicates poorer attention and more impulsiveness of response (Conners & Rothschild, 1968). The test took about 8 minutes, so it does not qualify as a test of *sustained* attention, but is more like a repeated match-to-sample test without a memory delay.

Factor Analysis

It is helpful to reduce the number of measures by factor analysis. Since several of the tests used are strongly influenced by age, each of the preceding variables was age-corrected by regressing age against all the

TABLE 3.1
Factor Analysis of Neuropsychological Tests

Variable	Perceptuo-motor	Achievement	Rote Learning	Attentiveness	Impulse Control
WISC Verbal	.59	.40	−.31	.13	.02
WISC Performance	.73	.09	−.27	−.08	.02
WRAT Reading	.10	.92	−.05	−.09	−.06
WRAT Spelling	.07	.92	−.07	−.14	−.07
WRAT Arithmetic	.18	.78	−.14	−.19	.04
Porteus IQ	.48	.19	−.14	−.31	.40
Porteus Q-Score	−.02	−.11	−.01	.09	.93
Draw-A-Man IQ	.70	.07	−.06	−.04	−.04
Bender-Gestalt	−.46	−.26	−.01	.51	−.10
Frostig PQ	.69	.01	.04	−.13	.01
PAL (Trials)	−.13	−.09	.93	.12	.02
PAL (Errors)	−.16	−.13	.87	.24	−.08
CPT (Commiss.)	−.06	−.02	.13	.79	.14
CPT (Omission)	−.05	−.29	.25	.63	−.07
Sum of Squares	2.38	2.70	1.91	1.55	1.09

SOURCE: From Conners (1975b). Reprinted with permission of the *Annals of the New York Academy of Sciences.*

variables and using the age-residualized scores in the analysis. The factor analysis of the entire battery is presented in Table 3.1. Factor I loads most heavily on visual-perceptual-motor tasks (Performance IQ, Draw-A-Man, Frostig Perceptual Quotient, Bender-Gestalt) as well as Porteus IQ and Verbal IQ. Although similar to a general IQ factor, one may interpret this factor as perhaps a bifrontal, right-hemisphere dependent set of tasks.

—Factor II is an academic achievement, Verbal IQ factor.
—Factor III is a rote-learning factor, showing almost exclusive loading by the paired-associate task.
—Factor IV is a combination of attentional performance (CPT), design-copying (Bender), and, to a lesser extent, Porteus IQ.
—Factor V we have called "motor impulse control" on the basis of the single loading of the Porteus Q-score.

Cluster Analysis

The above factor scores were submitted to a hierarchical clustering algorithm. In this procedure (utilized in our earlier discussions of symptom clustering), the program proceeds by combining the two subjects whose distance apart is smallest into one group, recalculating the distances between the remaining subjects and the new group centroid. This new matrix of distances is then searched for the smallest distance, and the two groups (or subjects) separated by this distance are combined. The matrix of distances is recalculated, and so on until the original set of N subjects has been combined (in N-1 steps) into a single group. At each step the increase in average within-group distance is computed and plotted. A plot of this value for each step in the grouping procedure yields useful information: A large jump in the value suggests that the level at which grouping is taking place has shifted; or, in other words, the groups combined at that step were more dissimilar than the groups combined at the previous step. Several such plateaus in the course of any one grouping run suggest a hierarchic structure.[3] Figure 3.2 presents the six profiles identified by the hierarchical cluster algorithm.

We have (perhaps somewhat audaciously) interpreted Cluster 1 as a group of children with "frontal lobe dysfunction." This is, of course, merely an hypothesis. The group is characterized by the lowest scores on the Porteus IQ, and the slightly lower general intelligence, poor Bender-Gestalt, Perceptual Quotient, Porteus Q score, and rote learning ability are consistent with deficits involving a bilateral frontal deficiency in these children.

Cluster 2 we have labeled "attention deficit/learning disability."(The poor achievement of these children may not be due to specific processing difficulties, but rather might be secondary to their attentional disturbance.)

Cluster 3 is apparently a group of children who have trouble following directions on the Porteus Mazes. Their tendency to impulsively dart into blind alleys and their forgetfulness in following the rules suggests a difficulty in the area of motor impulsivity.

Cluster 4 contains intelligent, high-achieving children who have deficits neither in attention nor in perceptual function. This is perhaps a group most resembling a "pure hyperactive" group *without* central nervous system dysfunction.

Cluster 5 is quite similar to cluster 4, but with a more striking facility on the CPT and rote learning tasks and less elevation of general IQ. This suggests a group of scrupulously attentive, cognitively intact children who may represent a population without learning or school problems but with problems mainly at home. They might therefore represent the most likely group in which to discover pathological family processes, poor parenting skills, or situational factors accounting for clinic referral.

Cluster 6 seems to be defined by poor visual-spatial abilities, but without accompanying attentional deficits. The moderately low

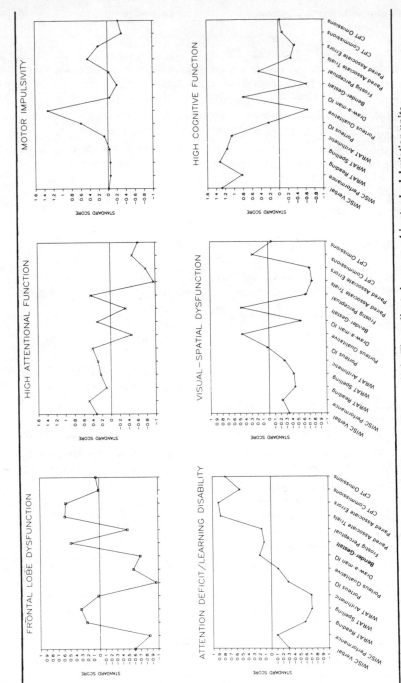

Figure 3.2. Neuropsychological profiles identified by cluster analysis. The ordinate is expressed in standard deviation units.

66

achievement suggests that this may be a "right hemisphere" impaired group with specific visual-spatial processing problems that interfere with learning.

In a previous publication (Conners, 1975b), we presented data on drug responsiveness, cortical evoked potentials, and motor development to illustrate some of the differences among these empirically defined cluster types. In Chapter 6 we will examine these clusters further from the point of view of their clinical significance in drug trials.

SUMMARY

This chapter has proposed the hypothesis that hyperkinetics as usually defined by clinical criteria comprise a heterogeneous diagnostic group made up of children who have at least four types of dysfunction related to two major brain systems: an inhibition system and an activation system. In addition, specific sensory and information-processing systems involving verbal and spatial information are closely intertwined with inhibitory and arousal systems of the brain.

Clinical neuropsychological evidence supports the existence of subtypes of children with problems of disinhibition, attentional/learning problems, and visual-spatial dysfunction, as well as children with quite intact CNS function who nevertheless are hyperactive.

The question naturally arises as to how these *behaviorally* defined subtypes relate to the *symptomatically* defined subtypes described earlier. Unfortunately, the data sets are largely nonoverlapping so we have not been able to do the logical comparisons that are indicated. We can only point to a certain parallelism and speculate that some of the symptomatic subtypes arise from deficits defined by certain of the neuropsychological subtypes. For example, the symptom complex of impulsive, hyperactive, moderately conduct-disordered children seems a logical candidate for "frontal lobe dysfunction." The highly attentive, obsessional and anxious symptomatic subtype might well overlap considerably with the highly attentive, noncognitively impaired subgroup identified by direct testing, and so on.

We do not press this issue because we regard both data sets as subject to important limitations and primarily useful as the basis for hypotheses. In particular, our studies of cluster analysis have the important limitation that some of the variables were age-standardized, and others such as the CPT and paired-associates tests, were not. This fact led us to regress out age variance in order to have comparability of measures across ages. But in so doing we may well have removed important information regarding those subtypes that represent maturational delays. In future studies cluster types will need to be identified within small age spans so that continuities and discontinuities in neuropsychological development can be properly distinguished.

We believe, however, that the data are supportive of our general hypotheses that brain-based subtypes can be identified among hyperkinetics, and at least two major dimensions of brain function underlie the behavioral phenotypes observed clinically. Future work that combines brain-imaging and neuropsychologic techniques will undoubtedly refine the suggestions made here of a link between specialized systems involving frontal-reticular-parietal loci and functions of inhibition, activation/attention, and spatial analysis. These new techniques of brain imaging already indicate that there is a significant role of frontal cortical systems in hyperkinesis and learning disorders; but they also make it clear that rather complex functional brain systems including other brain areas are also important.

NOTES

1. Dr. Karl Pribram provided us with the correct interpretation of these data in a debate on hyperkinesis at a recent meeting of the American Psychological Association.

2. We are indebted to Dr. C. T. Gualtieri and Robert Hicks for calling this paper to our attention.

3. Because it is sometimes alleged that different algorithms produce different cluster results, we subjected the same data to five other clustering procedures. The concordance across methods was extremely high, reassuring us that the resultant profiles represent some true structure in the data and not artifacts of the method. Contingency coefficients between the six methods ranged from .69 to .90 (Conners & Applebee, unpublished).

4

ATTENTION

In previous chapters we have emphasized the problem of heterogeneity among hyperkinetics, both at a symptomatic and a cognitive-neuropsychological level. We now examine the concept of "attention" that has often been proposed as a fundamental deficit in these children, and ask the question of whether and in what sense hyperkinetics may be said to have an attentional deficit.

ACTIVATION, ANTICIPATION, AND PREATTENTIVE PROCESSES

Resting Arousal

The hypothesis that hyperkinetics are deficient in arousal was first proposed by Satterfield and colleagues (Satterfield, Cantwell, & Satterfield, 1974). However, there is little evidence in the literature to support the notion that the "resting" arousal level of hyperkinetic children is different from normals (Hastings & Barkley, 1978). One obvious problem in studies of attentional tasks has been the heterogeneity of the patients who have been studied. Few studies attempt to control for subject characteristics that might affect response *other than the ones used to select the subjects.* Thus, as noted earlier, within a group of hyperkinetic children, some will show considerably higher anxiety levels than others, and if this factor is not controlled, it might well influence findings on arousal levels since higher levels of measures of anxiety will usually be associated with more autonomic and central reactivity.

For example, in their comparison of hyperactive and nonhyperactive learning-disabled children, Delamater, Lahey, and Drake (1981) found no autonomic differences between these groups in response to a task, but inspection of their rating scale data reveals that their hyperactive group was significantly more anxious than the nonhyperactive controls. In a reanalysis of these data (Delamater & Lahey, 1983), the subjects were divided according to their Conduct Disorder (CD) and Anxiety (A) factor scores in a 2×2 design. The results then showed that the high CD, low A subjects had significantly smaller skin conductance amplitudes and lower responsiveness than other groups. As expected, the high A subjects showed significantly increased heart rate. (Unfortunately, although the analysis shows that anxiety and conduct disorder interact, it does not address the question of how anxiety interacts with hyperactivity status, independent of the CD factor.)

Studies carried out in our laboratory with Eric Taylor (Conners, 1975a) addressed the issue of the confounding role of anxiety among hyperkinetic children. With anxious children included in the hyperkinetic sample, resting measures of arousal such as skin conductance (galvanic skin response, or GSR) showed no relationship to neurological soft signs or other indices of central nervous system dysfunction. However, with anxious children excluded, those hyperkinetics with abnormal soft signs had significantly less GSR activity during the pretask resting period compared with sibling controls (Conners, 1975a). Moreover, once hyperkinetic children who were clinically anxious were excluded, those with histories suggestive of CNS dysfunction could be perfectly discriminated from those with normal histories on the basis of skin conductance alone, indicating that heterogeneity in the degree of neurological involvement is also an important source of variance in measurement of arousal (and also incidentally suggesting that the GSR could serve as a useful diagnostic tool). Since higher anxiety level is associated with higher resting autonomic arousal, and neurological signs of CNS immaturity are associated with lower resting arousal level, differences in resting arousal between hyperkinetics and controls will depend upon how the samples are initially selected with respect to these variables.

This finding was confirmed by a study of Klove and Hole (1979), who compared 62 nonanxious hyperactive children with 12 hyperactives diagnosed as having anxiety-related psychologic disturbances and 10 normal controls. This is one of the few studies to select out the subgroup of "hyper-*reactive*" children carefully before examining the role of autonomic arousal. There were substantial differences in resting skin conductance levels between the two types, with the hyperactives having significantly lower baseline levels and lower spontaneous skin conductance activity than controls or anxious-hyperactives. Barkley and Jackson's (1977) conclusion that resting autonomic arousal is unimportant in hyperkinesis is based entirely upon studies that failed to subdivide the samples according to initial clinical state.

As in our study, Klove and Hole (1979) found that the nonanxious hyperactives had more signs of insult to the central nervous system. The low-arousal subjects had a high incidence of birth accidents, accident-proneness of a severe degree, and an excess of both high and low birth weights. This constellation of findings suggests that there exists a subgroup of children who are underaroused, and are also neurologically at risk, and another group who are anxious or excitable without neurologic signs or history suggestive of CNS insult. Mixing these groups has undoubtedly confounded any attempts to discover regularities in autonomic response patterns.

Task Arousal

When one gets ready to process a stimulus, a number of cortical and autonomic adjustments occur in anticipation of responding. These "preattentive" or "getting set" processes appear in several forms. Typically, the EEG shows a temporary blocking of rhythmic alpha activity and a slow negative shift (contingent negative variation, or CNV). Autonomic changes indicative of increased sympathetic tone occur (e.g., increase in heart rate), and these changes may vary as a function of the amount of effort or interest (Kahneman, 1973). Inhibitory responses such as vagally mediated heart rate deceleration occur (Lang, Ohmans & Simons, 1978) and there is usually a moment in which there is a generalized inhibition of motor activity, a "steady, unblinking eye" (Webb & Obrist, 1970) and an inhibition of spinal reflexes (Requin, 1969).

Both excitatory (arousal) and inhibitory preparations occur together in reciprocal and complementary fashion. These various preparatory responses are loosely coupled, and though each may independently affect performance, they probably represent overlapping but partially independent systems that come into play during different phases of the information-processing sequence. Thus, there is no single measure of "arousal" but a series of processes tied together by their role in preparation for "getting set" to respond efficiently. Under appropriate test conditions there are substantial differences between hyperkinetics and controls in autonomic responsiveness or phasic arousal during tasks. As seen in Figure 4.1, large differences in autonomic reactivity in a simple go-no go task were found between hyperkinetics, their normal siblings, and nonhyperactive clinic patients, with respect to both the latencies

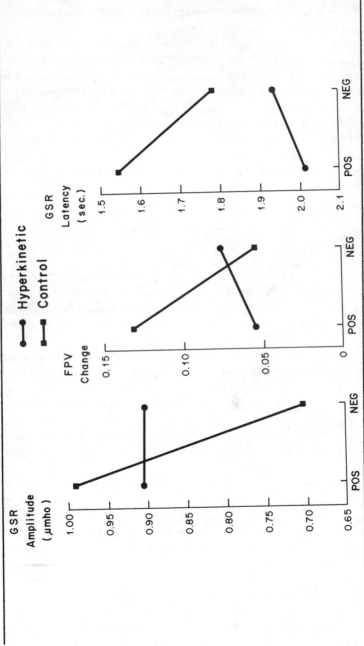

Figure 4.1. Galvanic skin response (GSR) and finger pulse volume (FPV) of hyperkinetics and sibling controls in a "go/no-go" discrimination task. The children must press a key for a high or low tone that is the go stimulus but must inhibit response to the no-go stimulus. Hyperkinetics show much less autonomic response to the two types of stimuli than do controls. From Conners (1975a, p. 163). Reprinted with permission of publisher.

and amplitudes of GSR and finger pulse volume (FPV). Again, this sample of hyperkinetics had been carefully screened to eliminate clinically anxious children. Children simply had to press a key when either a high tone or a low tone designated as the target occurred. As noted by others (Zahn, Abate, Little, & Wender, 1975), the hyperkinetics appear to have extremely sluggish or late-responding autonomic function. They appear to have difficulty in repeatedly "getting set" for the regularly occurring signals.

Inhibitory Processes

In addition to these differences between hyperkinetics and controls in "arousability" in task situations, they also demonstrate failure of *inhibition* of autonomic adjustments. In warned reaction time paradigms there is a typical triphasic cardiac response, with faster response associated with a greater cardiac deceleration. Hyperkinetic children do not show the expected relationship between speed of responding and cardiac deceleration during a warned reaction time paradigm. This relationship becomes normalized, however, following stimulant drug treatment (Sroufe et al., 1973; Porges & Smith, 1980; Portes, Walter, Korb, & Sprague, 1975). Cardiac deceleration is under control of a cholinergically mediated vagal inhibitory system. Control subjects also show a more *consistent* heart rate deceleration during the warning period than hyperactives. This inconsistency or lack of "fine tuning" of heart rate suggests an unstable central control system, not merely a permanently maladjusted level of responsiveness or activation.

In both our study (Conners, 1975a) and the study by Klove and Hole (1979), the GSR response of hyperkinetics also habituated more slowly to repeated tones than controls, a finding interpretable as a deficiency in developing appropriate inhibition over responses elicited by inconsequential stimuli.

ATTENTIONAL FUNCTION

William James must have been joking when he asserted, "Everyone knows what attention is." Perhaps a more appropriate view is, "Attention is not a single concept, but a complex field of study" (Posner, 1975, p. 475). In addition to the preattentive processes already mentioned, distinctions need to be made between *automatic* attentional processes, and attentional *effort* (Kahneman, 1973); and between stimulus and response aspects of *selectivity* in information processing.

Selective Attention

In most tasks involving attention to stimulus input, it is difficult to dissociate the phasic alerting processes just described from processes involving discrimination and selective attention to the relevant stimulus dimensions; in other words, the energetic as contrasted with the encoding aspects of attending. Recent behavioral studies that specifically examine selective attention processes cast doubt on the assumption that hyperkinetics have deficits in these processes (Sergeant & Scholten, 1983).[1] One approach to the study of this problem has been to examine changes in cortical evoked responses during attentional tasks. But the slow negative shifts and desynchronization of the background EEG during task arousal that reflect an effort to "get set" may mask any specific processes associated with stimulus selectivity (Naatanen, 1970).

One way out of this problem has been the use of the so-called oddball paradigm: If auditory stimuli are presented *rapidly* to the two ears, and subjects are required to attend to one ear, evoked potentials (EPs) to both the relevant target and irrelevant nontarget stimuli in the attended ear are enhanced relative to the unattended ear, suggesting a specific effect upon selective attention apart from phasic arousal processes. This effect occurs for an early negative component of the EP at about 100 msec (generally referred to as N100). In addition, a later positive component at about 300 msec (P300) is enhanced for the target stimuli, reflecting endogenous processes related to selective responding (Hillyard, Hink, Schwent, & Picton, 1973; Wilkinson & Lee, 1972). Not only are the physical parameters of the stimuli being analyzed more efficiently, but a particular subset of the attended stimuli is selectively attended to according to some predetermined rule (e.g., "this is a target"). The speed and difficulty of this dichotic task is supposed to allow measurement of the stimulus encoding activity uncontaminated by the slower phasic arousal processes occurring with each stimulus.

Some evoked potential data on this problem apparently support the notion that hyperkinetics do have a deficit in selective attention. Normal children show a considerable enhancement of N100 amplitudes under conditions of attending to one stimulus channel (increases of about 44%), while hyperkinetic boys show a much smaller enhancement (about 14%). The hyperkinetics also fail to show an enhancement of the P300 response for the target stimuli, whereas normal children have both a larger amplitude and longer latency of this component (Zambelli,

Stamm, Maitinsky, & Loiselle, 1977; Loiselle, Stamm, Maitinsky, & Whipple, 1980).[2]

Attentional Effort

While these electrophysiological data apparently support the notion that, as a group, hyperkinetic children show deficits in selecting or encoding information, there are other complicating factors to consider. Hyperkinetic children are often described by others as lazy. That is, they appear to lack the required degree of effort in attention-demanding tasks, and this lack of effort must obviously affect their performance, apart from any specific processing deficits they may have. However, it has been difficult to separate this effort component from attentional processes of selection and gating out of irrelevant stimuli.

There is some evidence to suggest that the *latency* of the N100 component of the evoked response reflects this effort (Callaway & Halliday, 1982). The amount of effort required in an attentional task can be varied by manipulating the difficulty of the task, by comparing active and passive attending tasks, or by automating the task through practice. In general, more automatic processes free the organism for strategic deployment of available resources requiring a conscious effort of attending, and more difficult tasks require more "effort." In most studies, however, hyperkinetics have *not* been found to differ from normals in the latency of the N100 component (Satterfield & Braley, 1977; Callaway & Halliday, 1982). Thus, if N100 latency reflects the effort involved in processing the physical characteristics of the stimuli, on the basis of current evidence hyperkinetics would not appear to be deficient in this component of attention.

On the other hand, there seems to be general agreement that hyperkinetics do show *faster* latencies for the P300 component. Since longer latencies of this component are associated with higher amplitudes and more accurate performance, the longer latency might be presumed to reflect the greater effort required to make a correct response. The P300, among other things, thus appears to reflect the speed-accuracy trade-off in processing information.

Klorman et al. (1981) found that for late positive components recorded at the vertex, normal children took about 62 msec longer on the average to process target than nontarget stimuli, whereas hyperkinetics spent about 58 msec *less* in processing the target stimuli. Similarly, Loiselle et al. (1980) found an increase of 47 msec for controls and a 24 msec decrease for hyperkinetics. It would appear from these data that the hyperkinetics are responding prematurely and less accurately, and this fact is reflected in their shorter-latency P300s.

But interpreted in this manner, there is a serious puzzle from these evoked potential studies. If one conceptualizes attention as a flow of information, starting with analysis of the physical properties of the stimulus and proceeding to decision processes involving response selection, then it seems reasonable to assume that more efficient encoding at earlier stages of the process would also influence subsequent response processes. This simple model predicts that, insofar as higher N100 amplitudes are related to degree of stimulus selection efficiency, one would expect a positive correlation between N100 and P300 amplitudes. (This is apparently the case for normals, because Loiselle et al. found a significant correlation, r = .48, between N100 and P300 amplitudes for normal boys.) This makes sense, for every time a stimulus is presented and accurately analyzed, one also ought to be more accurate in selecting the appropriate response, and this should be reflected in the larger P300. However, a *negative* correlation of –.56 was found for the hyperkinetic boys. If the hyperkinetics were less efficient in selecting information to be processed (i.e., had lower N100 amplitudes than controls), why is this correlated with a more efficient response selection process (higher P300 amplitude)? That is, why is the correlation negative? One would expect that the difficulty in selecting information would be reflected in a correlated difficulty in the response process.

To resolve this dilemma, one must recall how evoked potentials are measured. Because of the signal-to-noise problem in recording these small potentials, EEG responses to repeated stimuli are averaged over many epochs of EEG response to the stimuli. Negative-going potentials are averaged in with positive-going potentials occurring at the same poststimulus latencies, and the resultant waveform reflects this summation. An alternative explanation for the Loiselle et al. findings is that the combination of larger N100 and smaller P300 for the hyperkinetics has nothing to do with poorer *selective attention,* but is really due to a slow negative potential which overlaps the N100 component (thus elevating it), with this process continuing to the point where it overlaps the P300 wave, and then is averaged into the positive waveform (thus reducing it). That is, if a slow negative component reflecting "alerting" or task arousal to each stimulus failed to terminate promptly following the stimulus, and instead carried over into the P300 latency range, it would appear as a reduced amplitude component with a faster latency.

We have already seen that preattentive autonomic processes show greater inertia among hyperkinetics, both in getting started and in stopping. If the same thing happens to the EEG slow waves that occur in anticipation of processing information, then presumably normals are able to terminate the slow wave more rapidly, accounting for their apparent enhanced P300s compared with hyperkinetics. That is to say, *normals are able to adjust their response pattern to the changing demands of the task,* to inhibit the process of alerting to a signal when the signal has terminated, and not to overreact to subsequent stimuli that do not require a response. As we have noted, failure to inhibit a response once begun, and not to react appropriately to changing stimulus demands, is one of the hallmarks of the functions attributed to the frontal lobes.[3]

If it is true that a slow negative wave reflects the effort to analyze the physical features of the stimulus (or perhaps the effort in "getting set"), this slow wave should terminate earlier when feature detection is easy and be prolonged when it is difficult. A substantial body of data supports the conclusion that this is in fact the case. Naatanen (1982) has reviewed evidence suggesting that at least two such slow negativities occur during selective attention tasks. The first has a shorter onset latency and is modality specific, frequently overlapping the N100 wave and appearing to increase its amplitude, while the second negativity is a frontal component with a longer onset latency. The former is more concerned with target-stimulus feature analysis; the latter presumably reflects further processing once feature analysis has been completed.

It has been suggested that the earlier negative wave is indicative of a mismatch detector while the later one reflects continued selective rehearsal and maintenance of the attentional trace. These slow negativities are distinct from the relatively fixed N100 component and are sensitive to the intertrial intervals between stimuli, as well as the difficulty in discriminating the stimuli. At longer intertrial intervals the slow waves are maintained over a longer period, as also happens when the stimuli are more difficult to discriminate. (This is mainly true for the later occurring, frontal negativity.) Thus, the slow waves apparently reflect dynamic processes that adjust to the parameters of the task.

In Loiselle et al.'s (1980) experiment the interstimulus intervals varied randomly between 500 and 1500 msec. In the Klorman et al. (1979) studies the stimulus presentations were fixed at one per second, with a 200 msec stimulus duration. These intervals are sufficiently long that slow negativities superimposed upon the P300 response could account for the apparently reduced P300 amplitudes among hyperkinetics.

Developmental Aspects of Attention

Both the N100 and P300 amplitude components are known to change significantly with age in normal subjects. Almost all studies of hyperki-

netic children have included a broad age range from 5 years up. Important developmental changes in attention might therefore be masked in
studies in which age groups are combined across broad levels for hyperkinetics and controls. Figure 4.2 presents amplitude data for the N1-P2
component as presented by Satterfield and Braley (1977), and P300 data
as presented by Klorman et al. (1979).

One interpretation of these findings is that the normals appear to
have already reached their maximum level of development at an early
age, whereas the hyperkinetics start with smaller amplitudes and
develop more rapidly over this age range. If a maturational lag
hypothesis is invoked there is the embarrassment (at least in Satterfield
& Braley's data) that the hyperkinetics would seem to be *more mature* at
the older age levels than their normal counterparts. Callaway, Halliday,
and Naylor (1983) also concluded that a simple maturational lag
hypothesis cannot explain the evoked potential problems of
hyperactives.

However, interpretation of developmental changes in evoked potentials depends upon how valid the *cross-sectional* age data are as an
indication of *longitudinal* changes within the same subjects. There is no
guarantee that when the 6-year-olds reach adolescence their EPs will
look like the EPs of the adolescents in the cross-sectional data. Children
who are still hyperactive at age 16 may not be from the same pool as
children who are hyperactive when young but who continue to become
more normal with age. In fact this latter group of rapidly maturing
hyperkinetics would not find their way into the older age samples at all.
As a result, cross-sectional comparisons would be made between older
and younger children with fundamentally different disorders, or perhaps disorders differing greatly in severity.

The only longitudinal investigation of hyperkinetics that included
neurophysiological measures is provided by Satterfield and colleagues'
most recent follow-up of their original hyperactive and control samples
(Satterfield & Schell, 1984). They obtained court records for most of
their original hyperkinetic subjects who had been tested 8 years earlier.
They were then able to divide the groups in terms of delinquent and
nondelinquent outcomes using the criterion of felony arrests. Of the
hyperactives, 65 were classified as nondelinquent and 31 as delinquent.
There were 35 concurrent controls, none of whom had arrest records.
(The number of hyperactives who became felons is itself an amazing
statistic, made possible only by direct access to court records. Follow-up
interviews in other studies almost certainly underestimate delinquent
outcomes because of denial and falsification by the probands.)

The surprising outcome of this study was that all of the findings of
EEG and evoked response abnormality (as determined by comparison

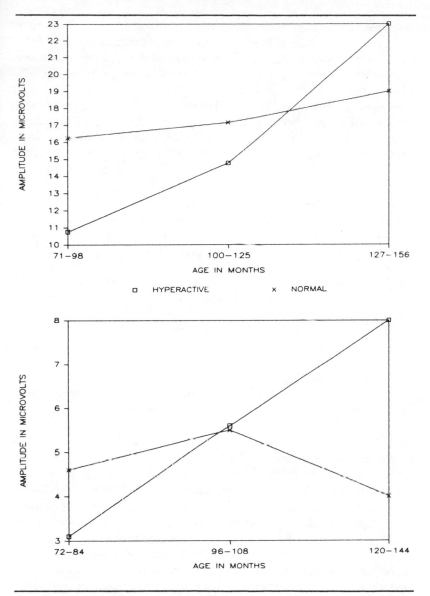

Figure 4.2. Event-related potential and age in hyperactive and normal subjects.
(a) N200 components as reported by Satterfield and Braley, 1977.
(b) P300 components as reported by Klorman et al., 1979.

with normal controls at the time the children were originally studied)
occurred in the *non*delinquent sample. Counterintuitively, the children
with normal evoked responses go on to become felons! The amplitude of
the N2 component of the evoked response was an especially good

predictor. Using only two-parent families (to control for the larger number of single-parent families among the delinquents), Satterfield reported that 50% of the hyperactives who went on to become delinquents fell into the upper third of the amplitude distribution of N2, whereas only 12% of the hyperactive-nondelinquents fell into the upper third of the distribution. Satterfield interprets small N2 components as an index of arousal because of evidence suggesting that N2 decreases under stimulation. Since high amplitude N2 waves are associated with low arousal levels, Satterfield and Schell thus conclude that the delinquents constitute a subgroup of hyperactives characterized by low arousal levels.

However, inasmuch as the original N2 amplitudes of the delinquents were not different from the normal control amplitudes, it follows that the delinquents are normo-aroused and that the remaining (nondelinquent) hyperactives were abnormally highly aroused. (This is a finding directly in contrast to Satterfield's earlier speculations of abnormally *low* arousal levels in hyperactives; Satterfield et al., 1974.) Moreover, it is hard to understand how the arousal levels of the delinquents can be *causally* related to their delinquency if their N2 components do not differ from normal controls. What really remains to be explained is why the nondelinquent hyperactives showed lower N2 amplitudes than normal (i.e., are more highly aroused).

A quite different interpretation of these data is possible. In Satterfield's experiments the children were supposed to pay attention to a cartoon presented on a television screen. The auditory signals that elicited the evoked responses were unattended, background stimuli. Presumably, then, a lower response amplitude to these background stimuli might reflect *the lack of effort in paying attention to the cartoon.* Under this interpretation, the delinquent hyperactives are those who successfully obey the rule to attend as directed, while the nondelinquent hyperactives are unable to keep focus on the cartoon, perhaps because they exert less effortful attention. By paying more attention to the background stimuli, their N2 amplitudes are reduced (more aroused).

A further alternative explanation is also possible. Satterfield's interpretation of the N2 component seems at odds with other interpretations that view larger N2 waves as associated with an orienting or "noticing" response. Snyder and Hillyard (1976) proposed that N2 amplitude reflects the operation of a mismatch detector signaling change in background stimuli, similar to Sokolov's neuronal model of the orienting response. Naatanen, Simpson, and Loveless (1982) also regard the N2 wave as reflecting a mismatch detector but see it as a passive reflection of noticing the physical deviance of a stimulus from repetitive stimuli that is insensitive to the meaning of the stimuli. Thus, higher N2 amplitude is viewed as indicative of a kind of automatic detector for noticing stimulus changes, irrespective of whether the changes are meaningful. (To complicate matters further, there may be two N2 waves, N2a and N2b, with one being an orienting response to physically deviant stimuli, the other an orienting response dependent upon the meaning of the stimulus; the latter might be part of the P300 complex and represent a higher-order analysis of the stimuli.)

According to this interpretation of N2, a higher amplitude reflects *more* attention to the background stimuli in Satterfield's paradigm. Following this line of reasoning, one would conclude that the nondelinquent hyperactives are simply less responsive to the background stimuli in the experiment—that is, *less* aroused.

Regardless of exactly what the evoked potential component is measuring in these experiments, these data illustrate the incontrovertible point that study samples of "hyperactives" are heterogeneous. With the benefit of hindsight, it appears that Satterfield's urban sample of hyperactive children initially contained a sizable percentage of "predelinquent" youngsters who had essentially normal brain function but abnormal environments. This conclusion is supported by the fact that the delinquent hyperactives had significantly elevated factor scores on the antisocial scales from both teachers and parents compared with the nondelinquent hyperactives at the time of initial study. Moreover, the delinquent hyperactives had a significantly higher *hyperactive* factor score on the parent scale than the nondelinquents, indicating that they were seen as more severe problems by their parents. Once again, selecting the sample on the basis of one dimension while ignoring others has led to the expected heterogeneity of the sample.

Commonly employed attention tests such as the CPT show a continuous development of efficient performance with age. Levy (1980) measured the CPT in normal children from 48 to 90 months and found that errors of omission declined almost linearly with age. Similarly, she found that motor inhibition, as measured by the draw-a-line-slowly test improved in near-linear fashion with age. By partialling out the common age effect it can be demonstrated that the correlation between the two tasks approaches unity. Thus attention and motor inhibition covary exactly across the age span in these cross-sectional data. The direction of causality is unclear, of course; success on either task could depend upon skills required in the other task, or each could be influenced by maturational processes common to both, or, as we suspect, CPT performance and voluntary motor control both depend upon the same fundamental processes of activation and inhibition.

SUMMARY

Focus upon the concept of attention has led investigators to look for problems in selectivity in attention, and to use the cortical evoked response as an index of such processes. However, careful examination of the experimental paradigms and empirical findings do not give unequivocal support to the notion of a selective attention deficit. In particular, the effortful component of attention, involving the ability to become appropriately alerted toward relevant stimulation, and inhibitory processes required to terminate processing once begun, have not been ruled out as explanations. Some hyperkinetics appear to suffer from deficiencies in alerting ("getting set" or being physically aroused to an appropriate level), and appropriately maintaining and terminating responses once begun. But baseline levels and task responsivity of central and autonomic indices appear to vary as a function of other variables, such as the level of anxiety, and how the sample is initially defined will partially determine whether the hyperactive children are under- or overaroused in resting and task situations. Failure to take into account sample heterogeneity has impeded understanding of central and autonomic characteristics that are intrinsic to hyperkinesis.

NOTES

1. J. Sergeant recently described an heroic experiment in which carefully selected hyperkinetics were persuaded to perform in a vigilance task over several hours. Their performance decrements over time were no different than matched controls, and their ability to attend selectively was unimpaired. What did distinguish them was the amount of effort required to keep them engaged in the task (personal communication).

2. In studies of hyperactives using the conventional CPT paradigm, concurrently recorded evoked potentials show smaller P300 amplitudes to the target stimuli (Klorman et al., 1979; Michael, Klorman, Salzman, Borgstedt, & Dainer, 1981). However, smaller P300 amplitudes during an active attending task are also found in *nonhyperactive* clinical groups, so the P300 results cannot be considered specific to hyperactives (Michael, Dainer, Klorman, Salzman, Hess, Davidson, & Michael, 1981; Dainer, et al., 1981; Lovrich & Stamm, 1983).

3. A number of years ago we noted that in the CPT, the increased errors of omission (often interpreted as a sign of inattentiveness) were actually a result of the fact that subjects were making many more errors of commission to the stimulus *following* the correct one (Conners & Rothschild, 1968). That is, their omission errors were really a result of responses that started too late and, once begun, could not be inhibited. Subsequent studies by Sykes and colleagues (Sykes, Douglas, & Morgenstern, 1973) showed a now well-replicated phenomenon that hyperactives do poorly in an experimenter-paced task compared to a self-paced task. We suggest that both the incorrect delayed responding (errors of commission) and increased omission errors on an experimenter-paced task reflect deficiencies in initiating and terminating a behavioral sequence.

5

MOTOR BEHAVIOR IN HYPERKINETIC CHILDREN

It has become fashionable to ignore motor behavior as a primary or core symptom of the hyperkinetic syndrome in favor of "attention deficit." Our arguments of the previous chapters will perhaps convey our conviction that this is a misguided effort. Having first defined their samples on the basis of parental referral for overactivity, investigators seem to have become preoccupied with finding everything else wrong with the patients but their activity patterns. Motor restlessness is, we believe, still the most important *symptomatic* characteristic of these children. Nevertheless, the deceptively simple concept of motor activity as a symptom also turns out to be rather more complex than appears at first glance.

THE CONCEPT OF ACTIVITY LEVEL

Gross motor behavior does not always distinguish hyperactives and normals, and sometimes one measure discriminates and another does not. These facts lead Whalen to conclude that some children show excessive motor activity while "still others may just seem unable to 'shut the motor off'" (1983, p. 164). This statement suggests that there may be different mechanisms influencing deviant motor discharge, with some hyperactive children having excessive activity level, while others have a failure of motor inhibition.

"Activity" has become a central concept in the understanding of both normal development and childhood psychopathology. Activity level at a given age, rate of development across the age span, and patterning of activity, are parameters that show important relationships with measures of personality, behavioral style, learning, and maladaptive functioning. Human activity, as in most mammalian species, is a recognizable trait with strong evidence of high heritability (Buss & Plomin, 1975; Buss, Plomin, & Willerman, 1973; Guilford & Zimmerman, 1956; Owen & Sines, 1970; Scarr, 1966; Schoenfeldt, 1968; Thurstone, 1951; Willerman, 1973). Activity level is also a stable and recognizable temperamental trait in babies (Thomas & Chess, 1977). It seems likely that biological variation alone will produce some children who are under- or overactive, traits that remain constant over much of the lifespan. These children are not necessarily abnormal, except in the statistical sense that they lie at the upper end of a normal continuum. Being an extreme case, however, certainly might predispose to maladjustment in an environment that does not tolerate excessive levels of motor activity.

But stable individual differences in activity level are one part of a more complex picture. One of the most fundamental facts about activity is its change with development during childhood years. Almost all methods of measuring activity show a decline of activity level with age, whether as a global impression of parents or caretakers, symptoms of hyperactivity, mechanical transducers of physical energy, or measures of the amount of space traversed in a standard area (Figure 5.1). Again, by general principles of behavioral ontogenesis, one can assume there will be pathologies of development involving a failure to modulate the level of activity in accordance with normative standards at a particular age. Such abnormalities may not reflect an intrinsically higher endowment of physical energy or need for movement as much as a failure to develop the increasing levels of control and inhibition required by the changing social expectations for the older child. Such control processes, as we have suggested earlier, may reflect fundamental aspects of brain organization and development. As with all biological substrates of behavior, many forms of insult may alter the competence and maturation of these control systems.

But activity is not merely a phenotypic expression of a genetic trait or simply an expression of built-in regulatory systems. The expression of activity is markedly affected by environmental variables that act to inhibit, exacerbate, or modulate the behavioral acts of the child—acts that are summed together by one method or another—and labeled activity. Activity in its broadest sense is a resultant vector derived from the social, educational, and perhaps nutritional environments interacting with the biological substrate of activity. The social environment creates a great variability in the degree and rate at which raw energy is expressed in overt behavior.

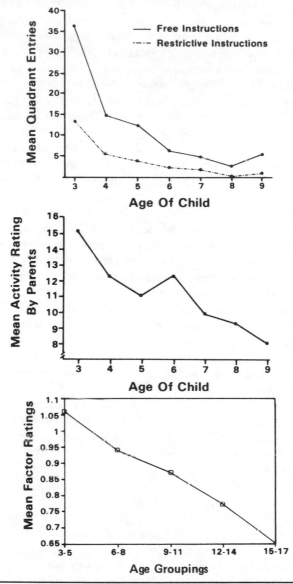

Figure 5.1. Changes in activity level as a function of age. (a) Grid crossings in standard playroom. (b) Parent ratings of activity level in various home settings as measured by the Werry-Weiss-Peters scale. From Routh et al., 1974. Reprinted with permission. (c) Parent ratings on the Hyperactivity factor from Conners Parent Rating Scale. Although all sources show decreases in activity level, the sources have low correlations with one another, suggesting that different types of developmental changes in activity level occur.

We may suppose, then, that there are pathologies of activity level that will be best described in terms of an abnormality of *pattern of fit* between environmental press and temperamentally based activity. For example, deviant socialization practices may lead to impulse disorders whose expression can resemble hypermotility. Such disorders are, of course, fundamentally different from impulse disorders that derive from the inability to apply restraint in the context of normally adequate socialization. Another type of "hyperactivity" is the profound curiosity that sometimes drives the talented child to continually challenge the bounds of boredom, perhaps incurring along the way the displeasure of some adult who finds him "hyperactive." How much stimulation the environment affords to such a child will clearly affect how hyperactive he appears.

At the other end of the continuum, the hypoactivity of the dreamy genius is not the same as the lethargy of the forlorn child. As with excessive activity, these are distinctions that can be made only as part of a pattern of findings involving both the child and the social environment; and for making such distinctions the human observer far surpasses mere quantitative recordings of changes in physical energy by means of the motion actometer or counts of small units of behavior.

Given these facts, it is not surprising that there should be disagreements among different operations for assessing the activity level. The human observer may not be as sensitive as a mechanical recorder in detecting energy expenditure, but the observer is sensitive to the meanings, goals, proprieties, and social codes that constrain behavior. The observer can detect when an event is a reward, a punishment, or a coercion and grasp the nature of physical or social pain that drives and constrains particular behaviors. The patterned appropriateness of activity is best judged by humans sensitive to the context in which motor acts are occurring. When the mother says her child is overactive, she may mean, "For me, in this house, at this time of my life, with my level of patience, and my expectations of behavior, this kid is overactive." Excellent, then, as a measure of the fit between behavior and the social context in which it occurs, such judgments may be meaningless with regard to pure quantitative measures of energy expenditure.

Mechanical measures make independent contribution to the prediction of behavior. It is perfectly appropriate to ask a parent whether their child is up and down at the dinner table a lot, but it is cultural norms that prescribe when a certain level of ambulation during dinner is too much, and it is these norms that also specify the sanctions that shape the expected behavior. The absolute level of energy consumption is only dimly related to many of these social variables. We may well expect to find, then, that correlations among measures of socially defined inappropriate activity and quantitative methods ("meter reading") of physical energy are low. Barkley and Ullman (1975) found that social and mechanical activity measures tended to correlate with each other, but the relationships were small in magnitude and differed according to the type of sample.

We believe the concept of activity level as a biological trait is quite meaningful, both as an independent and as a dependent variable. But judgments of risk-taking, drive, sensation-seeking, and curiosity behaviors may measure quite different dimensions of activity from high energy expenditure. Lack of restraint, or inhibitory capability, may not be the same thing as innately high drive level toward activity. The rubric of activity thus tends to obscure many distinguishable notions.

THE MEASUREMENT OF ACTIVITY

The measurement of activity is, unfortunately, a methodologic minefield. (Still one of the best reviews of measurement issues in activity level research, though slightly outdated, is the comprehensive chapter by Cromwell, Baumeister, & Hawkins, 1963.)

Rating and Self-Report Methods

Ratings are the method of choice when what is required is an estimate of the fit between the temperamental trait of activity level and the family. The Werry-Weiss-Peters Checklist (WWP) is an example of a rating method that has been successfully employed as a measure of home-based activity in a number of studies (Werry, 1968; Werry, Weiss, Douglas, & Martin, 1966). This scale records the impressions of parents regarding a child's activity in a number of settings, such as mealtime, television watching, play, sleep, and social settings. The scale has been factor analyzed (Routh, Schroeder, & O'Tuama, 1974), but there is little agreement between activity levels displayed in one home situation and those in another. Rated activity was found to show an almost perfect linear decrease in scores across the age range from 3 to 9 in normal children. Interparent agreement ranged from .16 to .58 (median = .33), and sex was nonsignificant as a variable.

The Conners teacher and parent rating scales each have a hyperactivity factor, both of which have proven drug-sensitive and diagnostically useful. Along with the 10-item abbreviated scale these methods have been extensively studied, and their ease of use makes them irresistible as "quickie" measures that allow comparison with a large normative database and many previous drug and diagnostic studies. But extensive use has also documented the variable and inconsistent relationship of such ratings to other methods, and findings are sensitive to context, informant, practice effects, age, and sex.

Ratings of traits such as energy, restlessness, fidgetiness, caution, aggressiveness, and assertiveness sometimes show strong relationships with level of activity as recorded by a mechanical actometer (Buss, Block, & Block, 1980). "Impulsiveness" is often linked with high activity level, but there are separate traits of venturesomeness (including risk-taking and sensation-seeking) and impulsiveness in speech (Eysenck, Easting, & Pearson, 1984).

Direct Observational Methods

Recording of free-field activity in playroom settings has provided valuable information regarding both normal and hyperactive children (Hutt & Hutt, 1970; Pope, 1970; Routh et al., 1974; Milich, 1984). Generally, these methods require that a room be marked off into grids from which crossings can be calculated. Routh et al. (1974) observed 140 normal children, 3 to 9 years of age, in a playroom divided into four quadrants. Each child was observed under instructions that allowed free play for 15 minutes, and also when they were instructed to restrict their activity to one quadrant. A systematic decrease in activity level was found in quadrant crossings with age, as well as a concomitant decrease in parent-rated activity level. Of interest is the fact that these two methods, though both showing decreases in activity over time, were uncorrelated. Thus, it was not the same children who were physically moving less and being viewed as being more socially appropriate.

Similar developmental effects have been shown for classroom activity using an interval-sampling method (Abikoff, Gittelman-Klein, & Klein, 1977). This method requires that trained observers count specific target behaviors within defined time intervals, a method that has been shown to be both valid and reliable in studies of hyperactive children (Abikoff, Gittelman, & Klein, 1980). These measures, however, do not always agree with other forms of rater judgment of activity, and in some cases are less drug-sensitive than the latter.

Mechanical Methods

Schulman and Reisman (1959) were among the first to apply the actometer to clinical child studies. The actometer is a wristwatch that has been modified to be sensitive to changes in acceleration. The validity of actometer measurement has been seriously questioned by Johnson (1971), who reported that when two actometers were attached to the wrist of someone using a hammer, the more distal actometer had significantly higher readings, suggesting that arm length may be a confounding variable. However, methodological studies have shown that arm length in young children shows no relation to results, and that although recordings from a single actometer are somewhat unreliable, reliability increases rapidly as more than one actometer is measured and several samples are recorded (Eaton, 1983).

Considerable data supports the validity of actometer measurement, though there are some conflicting data. Following a suggestion by Bell (1968), Halverson and Waldrop (1973) studied indoor and outdoor play activity in preschoolers, finding significant correlations across settings as well as significant relationships with teachers' ratings of activity. Importantly, the sex differences in activity were detected with the actometer but not with teacher ratings. Sex and age effects were found for staff ratings as well as actometer scores. Buss et al. (1980) found that actometer measures remained consistent across a 4-year age span. Stevens, Kupst, Suran, and Schulman (1978) also found that actometer scores correlated strongly with mother and trained clinical staff ratings of activity level. Milich (1984) found good intrasubject stability coefficients for actometers over a 2-year period, but only for restricted settings (r = .47) and not free play.

Kendall and Brophy (1981) examined the interrelationship of teachers' ratings (Conners Hyperactivity factor), a stabilimeter chair, and wrist actometers. The rating factor was significantly but modestly associated with the actometer (r = .26) but not with behavioral observations. The actometer correlated well with the stabilimeter (r = .65) and the behavior observations (r = .53). The stabilimeter also related well to the behavioral observations (r = .58).

ACTIVITY AND HYPERKINESIS

Gross Motor Behavior

It has often been argued that hyperkinetics are not globally more active but are more overactive than normals only in certain situations (Ross & Ross, 1982). Part of the difficulty in proving they are more active in all situations comes from the widely divergent properties of activity measurement systems (Pfadt & Tryon, 1983). Another problem is the intrinsic variability in activity observed by most investigators since the time Laufer and Denhoff first proposed that variability was an intrinsic feature of the syndrome. In order to demonstrate a sustained increase in activity level one must observe hyperactive children and controls across many different situations over a considerable period of time.

Only recently has adequate study of this problem been carried out (Porrino, et al., 1983). Hyperactive and normal boys were studied in 12 age- and classroom-matched pairs over a period of one week. Motor activity was recorded by a portable, solid-state accelerometer. This actometer uses a solid-state memory and allows continuous measurement over time, with readouts at selectable time intervals (Colburn, Smith, & Guarini, 1976). Parents and children also recorded a diary log of each hour's type of activity. Pervasive increases in simple motor behavior were found for hyperactives compared with controls across all situations, including sleep. There was also some situational interaction, however, because differences were larger for overall school activity than for other situations. Attentional performance on a continuous performance task (CPT) was an independent discriminator of the hyperactives and controls. The two groups could be discriminated with 87.5% accuracy using these two measures. The motor activity measure tended to misclassify older hyperactives (who moved less than younger ones), and the attentional measure misclassified younger subjects who had difficulty with the CPT. It appears that there are both situational and cross-situational differences between hyperactives and normals. However, the intrinsic variability of activity level makes it difficult to find such effects until activity is recorded continuously across many different situations.

These findings are theoretically quite important. The quantitative excess of activity during sleep for hyperactives is difficult to rationalize as the result of frequent attentional shifts or overreactivity to sensory input. Instead, it seems more compatible with an interpretation that mechanisms regulating inhibition of motor activity are deficient.

Using the grid-crossing method of measuring free-field activity, Routh and Schroeder (1976) showed that hyperactives performed like normals of a younger age. These developmental trends remain true whether the behavior is measured in free play or restricted situations, by means of actometers, grid crossings, or out-of-seat behaviors (Milich, 1984).

Fine Motor Development

Some hyperactive children are described as lithe, graceful, and precociously advanced in motor skills; others are seen as clumsy, uncoordinated and delayed in motor development. One frequently used assessment has been the presence of "soft neurological signs," including such tasks as rapid alternating hand movements (diodochinesia), visual tracking, motor overflow on one side of the body from activities initiated on the other side (mirror movements), jerky body, hand, or face movements (choreiform movements), and poor balance. A variety of methodological problems have beset the study of this area (Shafer, Shaffer, O'Connor, & Stokman, 1983).

Although individual items of this examination may be unstable, an overall index combining all items is quite reliable (Holden, Tarnowski, & Prinz, 1982; Mikkelsen, Brown, Minichiello, Millican, & Rapoport, 1982). Several studies have shown that these signs are more common among hyperactive than normal children or nonhyperactive clinic patients (Gillberg, Carlstrom, & Rasmussen, 1983; Mikkelsen et al., 1982; Werry et al., 1972). Since only about 50% of hyperactive children are reported to have soft signs (Casey, 1977; Kenny et al., 1971), they are obviously not diagnostic of the disorder. What, then, is their significance, if any? As in other types of motor behavior, these signs generally show a developmental course—disappearing as the child gets older— and are not related to any particular psychiatric syndrome (Rutter, Graham, & Yule, 1970; Shaffer, O'Connor, Shafer, & Prupis, 1983).

Because of the complex interrelationships among structures governing motor systems, it is generally not possible to localize the origin of particular soft signs (Lucas, 1980). However, there are neuropsychological implications of delayed motor development. By using converging information from psychological testing, neurophysiologic assessment, and neurological examination, one may infer some of the meaning of these developmental signs.

In one study (Conners, 1975b) we had a pediatric neurologist conduct a comprehensive neurological examination on 26 children, half of whom had low Verbal relative to high Performance Wechsler Intelligence Scale (WISC) scores, and half of whom had high Verbal relative to low Performance IQ. The two groups were equivalent in age (mean ages 9.6 and 10.2, respectively), and all had been diagnosed as being clinically hyperactive. The mean Verbal IQ for the high Verbal group was about 20 points higher than the low Verbal group, while the high Performance group had a 20 point advantage over the low Performance group. The neurologist examined the children without knowledge of their psychological test findings and used a total score on the neurological exam to divide the children into 5 degrees of soft sign impairment. The mean for the high Verbal, Low Performance group was 1.85 (SD = 1.5), and for the low Verbal, High Performance group was .54 (SD = .88). This difference is highly significant (t = 2.76, p = .01). The results indicate that the children with low Performance IQ relative to Verbal IQ are significantly more impaired on the neurological exam.

In this same study (Conners, 1975b) the children were asked to attend to the visual modality and make a response to an infrequently occurring dim flash amid a series of bright flashes. The EEG during the 500 msec following the bright flashes was averaged. The amplitude and latency of the largest negative-positive deflection between 100 and 300 msec was recorded. The results showed that the group with low Performance IQ had significantly smaller amplitudes and longer latencies of the N100 component. Moreover, the amplitude difference between left and right hemispheres was significant (t = 3.51, p < .01). This hemisphere discrepancy score is significantly correlated with degree of neurologic abnormality (r = .51, p < .01). Thus, children with minor neurologic abnormalities in this study seemed to be processing simple visual information more slowly and with less responsivity in the right than in the left hemisphere.

In addition to these differences, the low Performance group had Porteus Maze IQs almost 19 points lower than the high Performance IQ group, a difference that is highly significant (t = 3.07, p = .005). The low Performance group also showed more errors on the Porteus Qualitative score, which measures impulsivity, and failure to follow directions while solving the mazes (t = 2.05, p < .05). Thus, children with poor soft-sign neurologic exams appear to have deficits in right hemisphere visual-perceptual-motor skills and control over impulsivity.

We propose that poor motor development (as measured by this neurological examination), in association with impaired functions involving right hemisphere processing, constitutes a specific subtype among behaviorally defined hyperactive children. Rather than assuming that all hyperactive children are uniformly impaired in visual-motor perceptual functioning, these data suggest that some hyperactive children are characterized by a delay in cortical development, perhaps extending throughout the right hemisphere but certainly involving the motor and premotor areas, and possibly extending posteriorly past the central motor strip into the parietal association areas.

There is an important role of eye movements and movements of the body in three-dimensional space in the genesis of internal spatial coordinates (Rudel, 1982). Therefore, deficiencies in "visual perception" could arise quite independently of delays in parietal association areas related to perception, being of primarily motor origin. The constructional nature of most so-called visual perception tasks (such as picture arrangements, block designs, and Bender-Gestalt designs), means that voluntary movement is an important aspect of success on these tasks. (But by the same token, there is an important role of parietal cortex in visual attention to spatial information; see Bremner, 1982. Parietally based visual attentional functions cannot be ruled out as important contributors to performance on these tasks.) In all likelihood these systems mature together and interact over the course of development.

Others have also observed a relationship between soft signs, age, and psychological test performance. Mikkelsen et al. (1982) found that hyperactive boys had more soft signs than enuretic or normal controls; they also found a significant negative relationship between Performance IQ and soft signs (r = −.47) but not between Verbal IQ and soft signs. Soft signs were significantly associated with the presence of EEG abnormalities among the hyperactives (although this difference was confounded with age differences). This study also found a significant relationship with Bender Visual Gestalt Test performance (r = .51, p < .01).

Holden et al. (1982) reported strong relationships between soft neurological signs and the Object Assembly subtest of the WISC, arithmetic, as well as some weaker negative relationships with Performance and Verbal IQ. Another finding of interest was a significant correlation with the Learning Problem factor of our Parent Questionnaire, Hyperactivity, and Conduct problems, but not with Psychosomatic or Anxiety factors. Thus, minor neurologic impairment may have behavioral as well as cognitive correlates. Woods and Eby (1982) reported that aggressive, explosive child psychiatric inpatients had significantly more minor motor signs, including clumsiness, disdiodochinesis, choreiform movements of the extremities, and hypotonia. Excessive mirror movements significantly discriminated aggressive and nonaggressive children once the groups were equated for sex. They interpret the results to mean that aggressive and explosive boys have a defect of inhibition of inappropriate activity. In interpreting their findings, these authors note that the minor motor movements have an *intentional* character, and may reflect overflow of information between the left and right frontal cortices (Woods & Eby, 1982, p. 30).

Neuronal Excitability

Reflex responses of striate muscles are controlled by spinal alpha motoneurons. If pairs of stimuli are delivered at varying interpair intervals, a measure can be obtained of the rate at which motoneurons recover from stimulation. The recovery function typically shows that amplitude of the reflex is reduced with interpair intervals of 50 milliseconds, increased between intervals of 100 to 300 msec (secondary facilitation), and further depressed at intervals of 400 to 600 msec.

Pivik and Mercier (1979) showed in young adults that the secondary facilitation is significantly attenuated or absent during sleep. However, among hyperactive children, Mercier and Pivik (1983) found that secondary facilitation was virtually absent in both waking and sleeping stimulation. Hyperactives were also significantly more variable in excitability of the reflex at the longer intervals during the waking state. That is, instead of being completely recovered from stimulation after 5 seconds, there was great variability in neuronal excitability among the hyperactives. Recovery of excitability was much reduced among the hyperactives during wakefulness, and only one interval (100 msec) showed the expected reduction of excitability associated with sleep.

Mercier and Pivik examine possible neurophysiological mechanisms to account for the reduced excitability during the secondary facilitation period, since this period was the one most notably impaired among hyperactives. Because changes in secondary facilitation can occur as a result of feedback from spinal efferent gamma muscle interneuron spindles during the process of muscle relaxation, central cortical and reticular loops influencing spinal excitability need not be invoked as an explanation, though such explanations cannot be ruled out. In view of our earlier mentioned finding that habituation of spinal reflexes takes place in hyperkinetics at the same rate as for neurotics, we tend to favor a central regulatory mechanism as an explanation for the greater hyperexcitability of spinal motoneurones.

One interesting prediction that arises from the hypothesis that there is a general decrease in efferent gamma motoneuron excitability among hyperactives is that hyperactive children should actually improve when they are taught muscular relaxation. Increased central stimulation during relaxation of peripheral musculature could account for some of the paradoxical features of the psychophysiology of hyperactives in the literature. Centrally, they appear to be underaroused, insofar as their attentional and inhibition performances are diminished. Peripherally, however, they appear as tense and overreactive. Paradoxically, by relaxing these tense muscles, one should achieve an increase in central inflow from peripheral gamma efferent neurons, and hence an increased central arousal and frontal inhibition capability. We will further consider relaxation training in our discussion of treatment issues.

Once again, as with the results of the Porrino et al. (1983) study, the presence of abnormalities during sleep weakens the argument that hyperkinesis is simply a by-product of instability caused by poor stimulus control or lack of response to reinforcement contingencies in the environment; and argues instead that there are some persistent central nervous system abnormalities associated with the disorder. Whether and how much these abnormalities or motor excitability and recovery are specific is at present unknown because contrast groups of other psychiatric disorders have not been studied.

SUMMARY

In summary, at least some hyperkinetic children are characterized by subtle deficits in voluntarily initiated motor movements. Some also have slower motor development and decreased excitability of nerves at the spinal level. Subtle motor deficits are associated with psychological deficits generally thought to reflect right hemisphere information processing and voluntary motor programs involving the premotor and frontal association areas. These deficits are associated with smaller amplitudes and longer latencies in the right hemisphere for visually attended stimuli. Deficits of skilled movement can certainly arise secondary to poorer persistence and attentiveness (Humphries, Swanson, Kinsbourne, & Yiu, 1979; Schellekens, Scholten, & Kalverboer, 1983), but these factors cannot account for motor system abnormalities during sleep and across a variety of settings.

Since neurologic, perceptual-motor, and developmental motor skills are impaired in only a subset of diagnosed children, they probably represent only one dimension of brain function that can be impaired in hyperkinetic children. *Motor functions are themselves complex and do not represent a unitary behavioral dimension.* The cortical areas involved in these processes are interconnected and overlapping; and in the course of development, motor actions are required in order to contribute to the elaboration of perceptual systems.

The complex relationships among perceptual, motor, arousal, and inhibitory systems in the brain, and their mutual influence during brain development, make it highly unlikely that a simple primary activity deficit would be found among children. Failure to think of the problem from the perspective of the brain's structure and functional interrelationships has led to oversimplification in theorizing about hyperkinetic children. Although the symptom of activity level is no doubt the most salient of the features that bring these children to clinical attention, it seems unlikely on the face of it that such a symptom would result from any single influence within the brain.

6

DRUG TREATMENTS AND HYPERKINESIS

INTRODUCTION

Without doubt, the single most striking phenomenon of hyperkinetic children is their response to stimulant drugs. The effect is both immediate and obvious. Often within the first hour after treatment a perceptible change in handwriting, talking, motility, attending, planfulness and perception may be observed. Classroom teachers may notice improvement in deportment and academic productivity after a single dose. Parents will frequently report a marked reduction in troublesome sibling interactions, inappropriate activity, and noncompliance. Even peers can identify the calmer, more organized and cooperative behavior of stimulant-treated children.

Many well-conducted placebo-controlled studies attest to the efficacy of stimulants in altering behavior of hyperkinetics. Several comprehensive reviews are available (Barkley, 1977; Conners & Werry, 1979; Werry, 1978). Usually 70%-90% of hyperkinetic children are reported as improving on one or more measures in these group studies. Measures have included global clinical ratings, specific factors on rating scales, observed motoric activity, quantitative motor activity measures, skilled motor performance, cognitive and perceptual test performance, detection of speech in background noise, speech fluency, handwriting, EEG and evoked potentials, autonomic indices, mood, achievement drive, risk-taking, peer perceptions, and academic performance.

Despite these impressive effects of stimulant drugs with hyperkinetic children, the hope that the neuropharmacology of these agents would elucidate the fundamental nature of the disorder has not been realized.

Biochemical hypotheses based upon defects in catecholamine neuro-transmitter function have not been substantiated (Ross & Ross, 1982; Shaywitz, Shaywitz, Cohen, & Young, 1983; Ferguson & Rapoport, 1983). Nor has the stimulant drug effect been found to be specific to hyperkinesis (Rapoport et al., 1978; Taylor, 1983).

The wide array of improvements is actually an embarrassment of riches. The results are not always consistent from study to study. For example, although most studies report decreases in activity level, other studies do not (Millichap & Boldrey, 1967). Most studies report improvement in measures of attentiveness as measured by the CPT, but equally well-controlled studies do not (Conners & Taylor, 1980). Although most studies fail to find effects upon measures of academic performance such as reading, spelling, and arithmetic (Barkley, 1979; Barkley & Cunningham, 1978; Gadow, 1983), some well-designed studies find clear effects (Conners, Taylor, Meo, Kurtz, & Fournier, 1972; Weiss, Hechtman, Perlman, Hopkins, & Wener, 1979). No consistent predictors of drug responsiveness in hyperkinetic children have been found (Barkley, 1976; Sroufe, 1975).

It is always easy to invoke methodologic weaknesses as an explanation of conflicting experimental findings. Some of the drug studies do indeed suffer from methodologic weaknesses (Barkley, 1976). However, we believe that the difficulties are more than merely methodologic. Most studies suffer from a fundamental *conceptual* weakness: belief in a unitary mechanism of defect in the children and a corresponding assumption that drugs produce a unitary effect upon the brain and behavior. These "magic bullet" theories of drug action envision a specific brain target upon which the pharmacologic probe acts in a highly specific way. In contrast, from a neuropsychological point of view one would expect that various functional systems would interact with one another in complex ways under the influence of drugs, just as the neurotransmitter systems themselves are interlaced in complex fashion throughout the structures of the brain. In this chapter we propose the hypothesis that drug effects depend upon the particular pattern of neuropsychological deficits in the child, as well as the different actions of drugs at different doses and at different points in time.

A great deal has been learned regarding the metabolic pathways and mechanism of action of the stimulant drugs, but the story is both complex and incomplete. For example, although much of the theorizing regarding amphetamine and methylphenidate has centered on their effects upon the catecholamine system involving dopamine and norepinephrine pathways, cholinergic inhibitory effects of methylphenidate have been found in rat brains (Shih, Khachaturian, Barry, & Reisler, 1975). Porges (1976) is one of the few investigators to propose a possible cholinergically based role of inhibitory systems in hyperkinesis. At present there is no definitive evidence for the role of any one of the putative neurotransmitter systems as exclusive mediator of the drug effects in hyperkinesis. It is not possible to specify a particular pathway of drug action or a single biochemical "lesion" responsible for hyperkinesis. Even if a drug has direct actions upon only one neurotransmitter system, each system is complexly interactive with others, so that the chain of effects may ultimately involve several other systems.

This principle is true for behavioral systems as well. In fact, if it is the case, as we argued in previous chapters, that hyperkinetics comprise a diverse group of neuropsychologically impaired children, then they ought to respond to drugs differently according to the nature of their profiles. Since their neuropsychological profiles are presumably indicative of specific patterns of brain deficits, one might expect that children with certain profiles would be responsive to drugs, while others might not. Moreover, children with particular profiles may show drug responsiveness, but for quite different target symptoms or behaviors than for children with other patterns of deficit.

In this chapter we will examine separately the effect of stimulants upon symptomatic behaviors and neuropsychological measures using rating instruments and tests described in previous chapters. The data from several drug trials are pooled in order to provide sufficient numbers to detect both the subtypes of the disorder and the diverse types of change brought about by these drugs. The drug trials were generally comparable in most basic respects, including subject selection methods, class of drug (stimulants), dosage, and duration of treatment. In these trials drug effects were generally studied over an 8- to 12-week period. All children were randomly assigned, double blind, to drug or placebo. Ratings and tests were collected by examiners unaware of drug assignment.

Our interest here is not to argue the efficacy of stimulant drugs—a point we regard as well proven. Rather, it is to point out the complexity of the stimulant drug effect in hyperkinetic children. We also address the problems of dosage and time-action effects, arguing against the notion that there is a single optimal dosage or, indeed, a single type of child who responds to stimulant drugs.

STIMULANT EFFECTS ON
BEHAVIORAL SYMPTOMATOLOGY

Teacher Ratings

Many of the children in our large cluster-analytic study described earlier had been treated with stimulant drugs. It is of interest to examine how the drugs affect teachers' perceptions of child behavior according to the different cluster groupings defined by neuropsychological tests. The pre to post changes in teacher rating factor scores for the drug-treated children were compared with the changes shown by placebo-treated children. For each of the teacher rating factors a t-test was computed comparing drug versus placebo gains. These t-tests are displayed in Figure 6.1 for some of the groups (Groups 2 and 3 showed no drug effects and are therefore not plotted). As before, a t-value of approximately 2.0 indicates a significant difference at the 5% level.

Group 1 contains the children we previously hypothesized as having frontal lobe dysfunction on the basis of the pattern of intellectual dysfunction, including low Porteus Maze IQs. The drug effects upon classroom defiance (Def), hyperactivity (Hyp), and general psychopathology (Ind or index) are all highly significant in this group (p < .005). Inattention, anxiety, and sociability, on the other hand, are unaffected. This pattern of drug effects clearly indicates that this is a group of children who become less oppositional and more restrained. Unlike the other groups, drug response for this group appears most like that of the stereotypical "hyperkinetic child": a marked improvement in externalizing symptoms with no change or worsening in internalizing symptoms. One could argue, then, that this particular drug effect is one of primarily enhancing voluntary control or inhibition of action in a group of children whose fundamental deficit is precisely in the areas of self-control and voluntary restraint.

Group 2 contains the learning-disabled, inattentive children. They fail to show any teacher-rated improvement during the drug trial, suggesting either that teachers or the rating instrument are insensitive to any attentional or learning effects in the classroom. The reasons this might be so will be discussed below in relation to dosage and time parameters of drug management.

Group 3 contains children we previously described as having problems in motor impulsivity and following directions, based upon their relatively poor Porteus Q-scores. They also show no drug-related

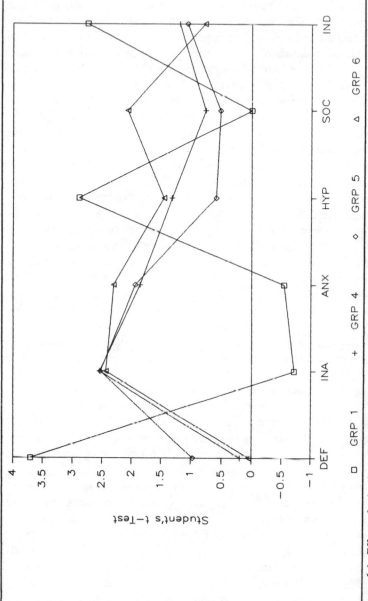

Figure 6.1. Effect of stimulant drug treatment on teacher ratings of behavior as a function of types derived from cluster analysis of neuro-psychological tests. Clusters are as described in Chapter 3. Abcissa are as in Figure 2.9. Two clusters without drug effects are not shown.

□ GRP 1   + GRP 4

+ GRP 2   ◇ GRP 5

△ GRP 3   △ GRP 6

improvement according to teachers. This is not surprising inasmuch as no items on the teacher scale would reflect this dimension of function.

Group 4 includes children we considered as having no particular cognitive deficit. They show strong improvement on teacher rated *inattention* and a trend toward improvement in *anxiety*. If one remembers that the items comprising the "inattention factor" of the teacher scale actually consist of daydreaming, social passivity, and "short attention span," then drug-related improvement on this factor is not surprising. This form of inattention is not really a cognitive deficit in the same sense as one usually applies the term to attentional deficits. It is rather the "dreamy" inattentiveness that accompanies withdrawal into fantasy and avoidance of social interactions. It is what English authors refer to as "unforthcomingness." The drug has apparently caused an increase in assertiveness for children who start as withdrawn and socially passive.

Group 5 we also characterized as containing children with no significant cognitive deficits, but unlike the previous group, they have relatively good attentional capability. Like the previous group they also show a stimulant-induced reduction of inattention and anxiety. Since these children are defined by their excellent performance on tests such as the CPT (which presumably taps some aspect of voluntary attention, resistance to boredom, or effortful attention), the inattention teachers rate as improving may reflect their perception that the children are less anxious and more able to perform task-related activities.

Finally, Group 6 is composed of children who show evidence of visual-spatial processing problems. They show significant differences between drug and placebo for inattention, anxiety, and sociability. (The apparent drug effect for the latter factor is actually due to a significant *worsening* in the placebo group rather than positive change in the drug group. One possible interpretation of this finding is that even though teachers did not see the drug-treated children as more sociable, they may have perceived a *worsening* in peer-related problem behaviors in the placebo-treated children compared with the stimulant-treated children.) Children with specific processing problems for visual-spatial information may also become more task-oriented and less anxious as a consequence of drug-related improvement in their cognitive function.

Though entirely post hoc, and therefore of hypothesis-generating value only, these results are certainly interesting in a number of respects: The substantial differences among groups in the pattern of teacher-rated drug changes, the significant drug influence on the psychopathology index (which is loaded with conduct as well as restless items), and changes in teacher-rated anxiety symptoms. These latter changes are rarely described in the drug treatment literature, and usually anxious children treated with stimulants are reported to get worse. However, some authors in the older drug literature have insisted that certain anxious, neurotic children show positive changes with stimulant treatment (see Conners & Werry, 1979, for a discussion of this issue). In contrast to the conventional wisdom regarding stimulant effects in hyperkinetics, the children most like a pure "attention-deficit" group show no drug changes at all, and the group with the least impaired profile (Group 5, "high cognitive function") shows substantial drug-related improvement. But the different groups change in response to drugs for different symptoms. Group 5, in fact, was shown to be the most placebo-responsive and least drug-responsive for certain tests such as the Porteus Mazes (Conners, 1975b).

These data are not definitive. The replicability of the clusters has not yet been tested, nor have the large number of separate drug treatment by group interactions been repeated. But the data provide strong initial presumptive evidence that various measures of function respond differentially to drugs, and such changes are a function of initial clinical profile. Not all of these children show equivalent drug-related changes, even though all met the initial (symptomatic) criteria for being considered hyperkinetic.

Parent Ratings

Figure 6.2 shows the comparison of parent factor score changes in the first four groups. (The numbers of ratings were too small for reasonable power in the other clusters. Indeed, the numbers are small enough here that power to detect effects will be extremely low, and these results are only minimally suggestive of effects that may occur with larger samples.) But a few points are worth making about the data.

First, the frontal lobe group again shows a significant effect for parent ratings of impulsivity, and this time there are also strong effects upon the hyperactivity factor and psychopathology "index" for the attention-deficit group. There is also significant drug-related improvement in antisocial behaviors in the group with motor impulsivity, a finding that is interesting in light of Porteus's claim that his Q-score is associated with antisocial behavior patterns. As is usually the case, drug effects on parent-rated behavior are weaker than comparable ratings done by teachers, and there is no consistent pattern of effects across the two sources of information. But even with these relatively limited data on parent reports, it is evident that the several clinical groups respond differently in the eyes of the parents. There is no simple reduction of attention or activity or impulsivity. Rather, the changes depend upon

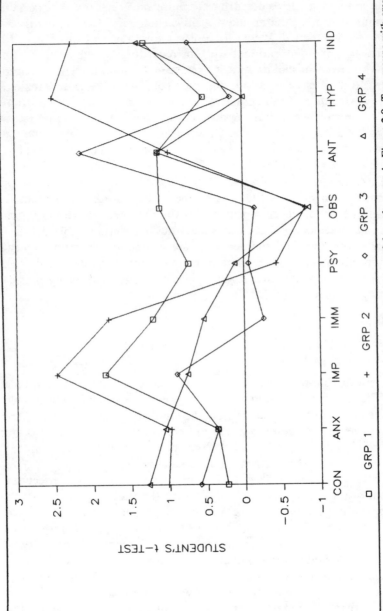

Figure 6.2. Stimulant drug effect on parent symptom ratings. Cluster type and legends are as in Figure 2.9. Two groups with small Ns are not shown.

the prior state of the subjects, as well as upon the particular behavioral dimension being used as a measure of drug response. More reliable response methods, such as standardized tests, give further insight into the issue of patterns of drug response.

PSYCHOLOGICAL TEST EFFECTS

We have previously reported that the Porteus Mazes shows signifi-cantly *poorer* improvement in Group 5 compared to all other groups (Conners, 1975b). While it is tempting to examine all of the test changes in this manner, there is a special problem in doing so: Since the groups are formed on the basis of these tests, the groups are by definition different in their initial levels for the various tests, and drug effects will be confounded with the law of initial values. That is, the clinical profile will be likely to show changes for those measures that have the highest score in the profile. A more appropriate examination of drug effects requires that changes be examined independent of the contribution of initial (baseline) levels of performance. Moreover, since the various tests are not independent of one another, changes among some of the tests will be correlated and one would like to know what independent predic-tors of drug effect are. Individual change scores are also quite unreliable and likely to produce an unstable pattern of results.

We handled this problem in the following way (Conners, 1972). We first intercorrelated the change scores on the tests and then factor analyzed the changes to produce "change factors." This procedure effectively aggregates changes that are correlated and produces factors whose reliability will exceed the reliabilities of individual change scores. We then used stepwise multiple regression with the change factors as the dependent (criterion) measures and the pretests as the predictors. Because the best predictors of the changes are usually the prescores most closely related to the highest loaded items in the change set, any addi-tional contribution of psychological tests beyond the initial level effects can be evaluated once these are accounted for. A subset of 178 drug-treated children had both pre- and posttest psychological measures.

Separate stepwise regressions were performed with each of the gain factors as the dependent variables. The results are presented in Table 6.1.

The first gain factor is largely the changes associated with the teacher questionnaire factors. (For this analysis we chose not to examine indi-vidual teacher factors; since one can argue that the scores are largely

TABLE 6.1

Prediction of Drug-Induced Changes (Factors) by Pretreatment Tests and Symptoms

		Weight	Gainers Are
Factor I: Teacher Ratings (multiple R = .73)			
Predicted by:	SQ Academic	.25	bad
	SQ Classroom	.31	bad
	Frostig PQ	.17	good
	SQ Authority	.26	bad
	WISC Performance IQ	.22	good
	Bender	.21	bad
	CPT Omissions	−.14	good
	Porteus IQ	−.11	bad
Factor II: Attention (multiple R = .82)			
Predicted by:	Paired Assoc. Errors	.59	bad
	CPT Omissions	.57	bad
	WRAT Arithmetic	.20	good
	WISC Performance IQ	.12	good
	PQ Hyperactive	.17	bad
	Drug	.11	On Ritalin
	CPT Commissions	−.11	good
Factor III: Perceptual (multiple R = .63)			
Predicted by:	Bender	.24	bad
	CPT Commissions	−.50	good
	Porteus IQ	−.36	bad
	Paired Assoc. Errors	−.25	good
	Porteus Q-Score	−.18	good
	CPT Omissions	.21	bad
	SQ Academic	.08	bad
Factor IV: Reading (multiple R = .58)			
Predicted by:	Age	.48	older
	PQ Neurotic	−.30	good
	Porteus Q-Score	.25	bad
	CPT Commissions	.31	bad
	CPT Omissions	−.19	good
	WISC Verbal IQ	.12	good
	SQ Classroom	−.19	good
	Frostig PQ	.11	good
	SQ Academic	.20	bad
	SQ Authority	−.15	good
	WRAT Reading	−.11	bad
Factor V (?): (multiple R = .70)			
Predicted by:	CPT Commissions	.44	bad
	WRAT Spelling	−.88	bad
	WRAT Arithmetic	.59	good
	CPT Omissions	−.43	good
	Porteus IQ	−.27	bad
	PQ Neurotic	−.20	good
	Age	−.39	younger

TABLE 6.1 Continued

	Weight	Gainers Are
Factor V: Continued		
WRAT Reading	.41	good
WISC Verbal IQ	−.11	bad
Bender	−.19	good
WISC Performance IQ	−.13	bad
Factor VI: (?): (multiple R = .57)		
Predicted by: SQ Authority	.47	bad
SQ Academic	−.38	good
DAP IQ	.23	good
WISC Performance IQ	−.22	bad
WISC Verbal IQ	.20	good
Bender	.24	bad
WRAT Arithmetic	.16	good
Porteus IQ	.08	good

NOTE: All regressions have an overall F-value significant at $< .005$.
Explanation: Weight = regression weight in stepwise regression equation. "Good" and "bad" refer to good and bad performance of few or more symptoms at pretreatment.
From Conners (1972). Courtesy of Charles C Thomas, Publisher, Springfield, IL.

source determined anyway, with teacher factors correlating most highly with themselves, we summed items across the three major headings of the teacher questionnaire: academic performance, classroom behavior, and response to authority.) As expected, the strongest predictors of these changes are the prescores for academic and classroom behavior ratings. As in much other drug work there is a strong rate dependency of drug effect associated with the predrug status of the subjects. But note also that measures of visual perception (Frostig Perceptual Quotient, WISC Performance IQ) are significant *independent* predictors of drug changes on teacher ratings.

Speculating here, one might suggest that the relatively good predrug status on these perceptual measures as well as on CPT omissions suggests that improvers on this factor are children who have relatively good right hemisphere function and attentional capability, and that their poor Bender and Porteus performance is consistent with poor planning and lack of forethought. In accord with our previous conclusions for Group I changes in parent and teacher ratings, a plausible hypothesis is that this first drug effect reflects changes in a subgroup with anterior frontal lobe dysfunction.

The second gain factor is for CPT omissions and paired-associate learning errors, clearly suggestive of changes in attentional function. Improvers for this factor are children who are both inattentive and hyperactive (according to parents). This is the most predictable of the drug-change effects (multiple R = .82). Again, the best "predictors" are the prescores on the tests defining the factor; children who are inattentive become more attentive following drug treatment. Higher prescores on arithmetic and Performance IQ also contribute significantly to the prediction, perhaps indicating that although the children are inattentive and hyperactive, they are quite unimpaired in functions involving perceptual differentiation and calculation; that is, in right hemisphere parietally based activity.

Gain Factor 3 we consider to be a motor impulsivity factor, involving as it does changes in CPT errors of commission, Porteus Q-score, and Porteus IQ. Low Bender errors were also strongly loaded on the factor, suggesting that it measures impulsiveness *without* deficits in constructional praxis. Since gainers on this factor were predicted by poor predrug status on CPT omissions as well, the results indicate that it is inattentive impulsive children who are changing under the drug's influence.

Gain Factor 4 we described as a reading factor because the most highly loaded item on the change factor was improvement on the WRAT reading test. Children who improve in reading tend to be older, nonneurotic children who have good WISC Verbal IQs and Perceptual Quotients, are not defiant in the classroom, but make many errors of commission.

Gain Factor 5 might be considered either a spelling or arithmetic factor, though changes for these two measures go in opposite directions. Improvers in spelling tend not to change in arithmetic and vice versa. Children who change on this factor are younger, more impulsive (high CPT commissions, low Porteus IQ), and have relatively low Verbal and Performance IQs. The pattern of changes is suggestive of a group of young, impulsive children who benefit from the drugs because their impulsive behavior is improved.

Gain Factor 6 is largely defined by two variables: drawings of a man and sound blending skills. We have previously reported that stimulant drugs have a significant effect upon human figure drawings (Conners, 1971). The prediction equation for Gain Factor 6 shows that changes in figure drawings are predicted by defiance in school, good WISC Verbal IQ but poor Performance IQ, and poor Bender scores. These children are also rated by teachers as having good *academic* performance. Perhaps these improvers are children with poor right hemisphere function but good left hemisphere function who are able to perform well academically despite their defiant behavior.

Several points should be made about these findings. First, we note that individual test scores by themselves are hard to interpret. We have stressed that it is the *pattern* of scores defining the subgroups that is important for understanding the drug effects. Similarly, *changes* in test scores are better understood when seen as part of a pattern of changes than as discrete measures of one function.

Patterns of change appear to be associated with particular patterns of deficits prior to drug treatment, though no simple generalizations regarding drug effects are warranted by the data. Changes do appear to be dependent upon the functional neuropsychological organization of the children, but it is not always easy to see just why certain changes are occurring for particular children. Nevertheless, the main message of interest to us at the moment is the futility of looking for unitary predictors of drug effect.

We are fully aware that the findings are limited by the particular battery of tests employed here. We have somewhat freely speculated about the meanings of our test findings and expect that we would have to modify our conclusions if a more representative neuropsychological test battery were chosen. For the moment we regard these explorations as a basis for hypotheses to be tested more rigorously on other samples with a test battery more theoretically constructed to assess specific processing and behavioral dysfunctions.

We regard it as proven that sample heterogeneity in neuropsychological functioning affects drug response. Much of the contradiction in the literature regarding drug effects comes from oversimplifying both the "diagnosis" of the subject sample and the diversity of possible drug effects.

DRUG DOSAGE AND
TIME-ACTION EFFECTS

A great deal of research on stimulant drug effects with hyperkinetic children has shown the importance of drug dosage as a variable affecting outcome. Sprague and colleagues (Sprague & Sleator, 1976, 1977) were the first to point out that dosages that are optimal for motor behavior and social behavior may not be optimal for cognitive behavior. What is the neuropsychological basis for the diverse dosage effects upon different behaviors? We suggest that stimulants affect more than one functional brain system, producing different effects upon response systems. This assertion is supported by observations of how stimulants act over time and at different dosage levels.

We carried out the following experiment (Solanto & Conners, 1982). Ten hyperkinetic children were examined under three different dosages of methylphenidate (MPH): .3, .6, and 1.0 mg/kg. Placebo was given on two other days, distributed randomly among the active drug days, and given in a double-blind fashion. Each session on a particular day included a baseline (predrug) session, during which measures of performance and physiological responses were taken, followed by drug administration and hourly measures of performance and physiological responding over the next four hours.

Each test session on a given day consisted of four phases: a 5-minute resting phase, passive listening to a repeated tone, and a serial warned reaction time test with a fixed foreperiod warning interval. Behavioral measures consisted of errors of omission and commission, reaction time, and seat activity recorded from a chair that counted seat rotations, tilting, and feet movement. Physiological measures included digital finger temperature, heart rate, GSR, and EMG (electromyogram). Figure 6.3 shows the dosage and time effects upon heart rate, errors of commission, skin temperature, and activity level.

The drug reached its peak effect within one hour at all dosages and then sharply declined to baseline levels within two to three hours. Similar findings were obtained for reaction time, heart rate, and GSR. The effects upon activity level were quite different, however. Figure 6.3(c) indicates that although the low and medium doses show a tendency to return to baseline as did the other measures, activity level in the high dose continues to decline throughout the testing day. Thus, there is an interaction between dosage, time, and type of response system.

We interpreted these findings as consistent with *two different physiological mechanisms* of drug action, having different dose-time-action characteristics. The faster-acting autonomic and "attentional" responses could reflect the impact of MPH upon thalamic and reticular pathways, particularly the thalamic and limbic centers, which regulate attention and autonomic response; while the longer-acting motor effects could reflect more anterior frontal lobe inhibitory effects operating somewhat independently of (and subsequent to) the arousal effects. (Alternatively, the different effects of low and high drug dosages could reflect different metabolic pathways that are engaged by the saturation of one system and overflow into another, a principle of pharmacodynamics that is well-known.)

Several implications of these findings seem apparent. First, the "window" of drug action is highly limited for the attentional effects. Obviously, any drug treatment of academic or cognitive deficits must take into account this narrow window of action. Drug studies that report failure of drug effects upon academic functioning invariably fail to specify the time-action course of the effects, often measuring the academic variable at some unspecified time during the day (see Pelham, 1983, for an excellent review of this and related methodologic issues in

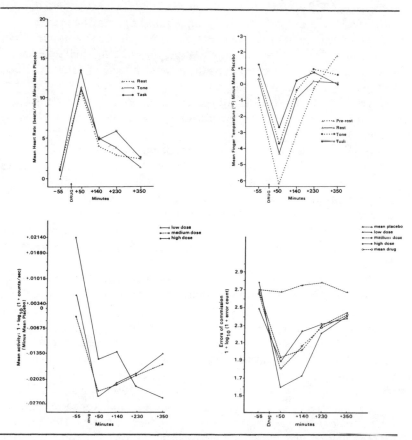

Figure 6.3. Autonomic and behavioral effects over time at three different dosage levels of Ritalin (methylphenidate) for hyperactive children. Note how high dose causes continued suppression of activity level, whereas attentional and autonomic measures show rapid return to baseline within about two hours. From Solanto and Conners (1981). Reprinted with permission.

drug studies of academic functioning). The fact that parent-rated changes are ususally based upon behavior long after the last dose of medication at school means that physicians who use parent report as the basis of titrating drug dosage will increase the dose to relatively high levels. According to our results, this will ensure a prolonged reduction in activity level. But early positive effects upon attentional function at lower doses may be obscured, perhaps overmedicating the children with respect to academic target symptoms.

Sprague and colleagues have argued that about .3 mg of MPH is optimal for cognitive functions, but in our study we found a linear increase in CPT performance with increasing dose. One explanation of the difference in outcome from Sprague's findings may have to do with the cognitive load imposed by the tasks used in the two experiments. In our study the attentional task was relatively easy, being in effect a simple serial reaction time task, whereas the adverse effects of drug described by Sprague involved higher cognitive load in a memory task. Thus, both the type of task and its difficulty level may interact with drug dosage. Therefore, no simple generalization about *the* optimal dose level can be made.

The clinical implications of this approach are important. Clinicians cannot use group drug studies as guides to therapy when these studies are composed of heterogeneous types of children. No good predictors of drug responsiveness have been found among hyperkinetics as typically defined, but predictions are quite good for individual subtypes. It seems plausible that different brain mechanisms must mediate different behavioral response systems, and that drugs will influence these systems in different ways at different times.

Clinicians desiring to establish the optimal dose of stimulant drug for a particular child must consider which of the possible response systems is the target, since dose-response varies as a function of the system being observed. Apparently, as seen in our data, the time-action effects of drugs also varies for different response systems, and therefore the optimal time of treatment will depend upon the particular target system. In particular, tasks requiring alertness and persistence, such as repetitive vigilance tasks, have a very narrow time window of drug sensitivity. Changes in gross motor behavior, on the other hand, appear to be more long-lived but require a higher dose to achieve this effect. Optimal drug therapy will require much greater precision in the specification of the pattern of deficits in the child, the target behaviors to be treated, and the time at which the crucial behaviors are likely to be exhibited.

7

INFLUENCE OF THE SOCIAL ENVIRONMENT

INTRODUCTION

Based on the data and formulations presented in the preceding chapters, we believe that a neuropsychological model best accounts for the primary symptoms of the hyperkinetic syndrome. Several subtypes of the disorder are derived from the combination of under- or overarousal and under- or overinhibition, which in turn may reflect extremes of function in frontal and thalamic-reticular systems of the brain. Processing deficits (learning disorders), which are frequent accompaniments of the various subtypes, may reflect dysfunctions in specific verbal or spatial cortical processors.

In addition to the primary symptoms, there are important secondary consequences of these fundamental brain-based disorders. We have emphasized that the social environment interacts with the child's deficits in a complex fashion to exacerbate, modulate, and pattern the child's symptoms. In other cases social factors can act as mitigating agents in children otherwise at high biological risk. Our view that social factors can act as accelerator or suppressor variables for children who are biologically or constitutionally predisposed to hyperkinesis is consistent with that of other researchers who have recently shifted away from an exclusive child-deficit model (e.g., Lambert & Hartsough, 1984; Whalen, 1983). In this chapter we shall attempt to present some of the research findings that bear on this question.

SECONDARY SYMPTOMS AND
FAMILY PROCESS

Aggression and Self-Esteem

The most direct and influential work in this area has been performed by Jan Loney and her associates. These investigators have made a distinction between primary or core symptoms of hyperkinesis (i.e., hyperactivity, inattention) and the secondary symptoms (i.e., aggressive and/or antisocial behavior; self-esteem deficits). Their research has strongly suggested that the primary and secondary symptoms are subject to different etiological influences, respond to treatment differently, and follow a different long-term course.

In the first of a series of papers on this subject, Paternite, Loney, and Langhorne (1976) examined the relationship among presenting symptomatology, socioeconomic status (SES), and parenting styles in 113 clinic-referred children diagnosed with hyperkinetic impulse disorder. The research staff made severity ratings for each of six primary symptoms (hyperactivity, fidgetiness, inattention, judgment deficits, negative affect, uncoordination) and three secondary symptoms (aggression, self-control deficits, self-esteem deficits) for every child. SES indices were computed for all families. Several parent variables were also examined using parent self-report, spouse report, and staff ratings of each parent along nine global parenting dimensions.

Results of the study showed different patterns of relationship of social and parenting variables to the primary versus the secondary symptoms of hyperkinetic syndrome. High and low SES groups differed on each of the three secondary symptoms, with boys from high SES homes showing less severe secondary symptomatology. In contrast, no SES differences were found for any of the six primary symptoms, with boys from high and low SES backgrounds showing equivalent severity ratings for primary symptoms.

Also of interest, differences between SES groups were found for several parenting variables. According to Paternite et al. (1976), "the general picture that emerges from the parenting data is of low SES parents who are more lax, easy-going, and inconsistent than are the high SES parents." Parenting attitudes and styles, particularly with respect to firmness and consistency, appear to vary as a function of SES.

Furthermore, in examining the relative contribution of SES and parenting to secondary symptom severity ratings, the most important independent predictors were parenting variables rather than SES (see Table 7.1). For the secondary symptom, aggressive interpersonal behav-

TABLE 7.1
Environmental Predictors of Secondary Symptomatology
in Hyperkinetic Syndrome

Child Symptom	Predictor
Aggressive interpersonal behavior	1. Father's hostility
	2. Mother too short-tempered
	3. Mother's inconsistency
	4. Mother's shortcoming
	5. SES
	6. Mother too easy going
	7. Mother autonomy/control
Impulse control deficits	1. Mother inconsistency
	2. Father's placidity
	3. Mother too short-tempered
Self-esteem deficits	1. Father's inconsistency
	2. Mother too strict
	3. Mother firmness
	4. Mother too easy going

SOURCE: From Paternite et al. (1976). Used with permission.

ior, however, the addition of the SES index variable did add significantly to the prediction.

Since the publication of the 1976 article, Paternite and Loney (1980) have replicated and extended their study of the differential relationship of social and environmental influences to the primary and secondary symptoms of hyperkinetic syndrome. Their second study included 99 boys from the full range of SES backgrounds, diagnosed with hyperkinetic impulse disorder, and treated with either Ritalin or dexedrine.

In examining the relationships among various factors reflecting home and environmental influences and primary and secondary symptoms of hyperkinesis, it was again demonstrated that relationships vary for different types or classes of symptoms. To begin with, *no environmental predictors were identified for the primary or core symptoms of hyperkinetic syndrome at referral.* In contrast, five environmental factors contributed significantly to the predictor equations for the secondary symptom, aggression. These predictors for the child's aggression, as rated by parents, were poor parent-child relationship, father too short-tempered, urban residence, parents-too-busy, and SES. For staff-rated child aggression, significant predictors were parental psychopathology, parent-child relationship, and mother-father relationship.

The research of Loney and her colleagues has been influential in showing that the secondary symptoms of hyperkinesis (particularly aggression) are strongly influenced by the social environment. That is, "Children who vary very little in age, I.Q., or primary symptomatology do differ in secondary symptomatology depending upon the nature and quality of parenting styles" (Paternite & Loney, 1976, p. 299).

Secondary Symptoms and SES

Loney's research has also demonstrated the importance of specifying the relevant controlling variables that are subsumed by the global factor SES. She and others have suggested that SES is simply a shorthand term for a conglomerate of complexly interrelated factors that should be studied singly and in combination. It is not SES per se that somehow exerts control over children's behavior; rather, the parenting styles, attitudes and practices, and other specific environmental influences that are correlated with SES are the more direct controlling influences.

Lee Robins (1979) reached a similar conclusion in her recent review of the epidemiology of aggressive behavior. She concluded that the effects of SES on aggressive child behavior are actually attributable to processes within the family. For example, in studies holding social class constant and examining differences between parents of delinquents and nondelinquents, parents of delinquents have been found to be less adequate in terms of overall social adjustment. They are less educated, make less use of available health services, and show less ability to obtain and hold a job. According to Robins (1979), because of their poorer social coping abilities these individuals are more likely to show poorer parenting abilities which directly result in aggressive child behavior.

Secondary Symptoms at Follow-Up

Other researchers have also documented a relationship between family ecological variables, secondary symptomatology, and long-term outcome. One of the most substantial of these studies is the Kauai longitudinal study, a prospective 18-year follow-up of all births in 1955 on the Hawaiian Island of Kauai as well as a selected sample of children considered "at risk" for MBD because of perinatal complications (Werner, 1980). All of these children were rated for the absence, presence, and severity of perinatal complications as well as the quality of the child's environment at 1, 2, and 10 years. By age 10, 3% of the total sample had been diagnosed as probably MBD with learning disabilities.

Importantly, there was a significant interaction between family environmental effects and perinatal complications. Among children who experienced perinatal complications that might be presumed to lead to MBD (such as anoxia, prematurity, and other obstetrical complications), the highest proportion with serious mental health problems at age 10 came from homes that were unstructured and disorganized in early childhood. In contrast, the rate of serious mental health problems among children with similar perinatal complications but who grew up in stable homes was much smaller.

In addition, at age 10, ratings of emotional support were made on the basis of the interpersonal relationship between parents and child, the kind and amount of reinforcement used, the methods of discipline, the ways of expressing affection and approval, and on opportunities provided for appropriate sex-role identification. Ratings of "high emotional support," clearly reflecting parenting and family management practices, were associated with the lowest rates of behavior problems at age 10.

Montreal Follow-Up Studies

Additional evidence for the influence of the family and social environments in hyperkinetic syndrome comes from the long-term follow-up studies of Gabrielle Weiss and her colleagues in Montreal. This research group has followed several groups of hyperkinetic children, initially evaluated in their clinic, to adolescence and young adulthood.

In one of their first reports, Weiss, Minde, Werry, Douglas, and Nemeth (1971) developed a rating scale for family competence. This scale consists of six items measuring marital relationship, child rearing practices, maternal deprivation, mother-child relationship, psychiatric illness in the parents, and socioeconomic status, with each item rated by a child psychiatrist on a 5-point scale.

At five-year follow-up, those children displaying overt antisocial behavior differed from the rest of the group by having had significantly higher aggression scores at initial evaluation and in having families who had been rated as significantly more pathological. Poor mother-child relationships, poor mental health of parents, and punitive child-rearing practices were the items found to significantly discriminate the families of the ultimately aggressive children from the rest of the group. In a later study, Weiss, Kruger, Danielson, and Elman (1975) reported that among a group of hyperkinetic children treated with MPH, family competence was significantly related to academic achievement, positive emotional adjustment, and the absence of overt aggressive behavior at follow-up.

The most recent study from the Montreal research group reported the 12-year follow-up data on the initial group of hyperactive children studied by these researchers (Hechtman, Weiss, Perlman, & Amsel, 1984). These children are now young adults, 17-24 years of age. Results of this study indicate that as these individuals mature, outcome is predicted best by the complex interaction of several variables. As in previous studies, socioeconomic status and the mental health of parents continue to be among the most important predictor variables.

Summary

To summarize studies on the relationship of the social environment to hyperkinesis, it appears that environmental influences are differentially related to the primary and secondary features of the syndrome at referral and at follow-up. At referral, the primary symptoms of hyperkinesis (i.e., inattention, hyperactive motor behavior) show very little relationship to environmental variables. This finding strengthens the supposition that the primary symptoms are endogenous, or related to aspects of brain development and function. In contrast, the secondary symptoms, notably aggression, are systematically related to parenting and family management practices and to SES.

The parenting practices most often related to secondary symptomatology have to do with hostile, angry parent-child interaction patterns and to faulty disciplinary practices. The latter are characterized by laxity and leniency in setting clear-cut expectations and consequences for child behavior and by the use of overly punitive or violent punishment. Parental disturbance and urban residence have also been related to the aggressive dimension of hyperkinetic syndrome. The consistency between these data and those collected by Gerald Patterson (1983), working with a purely aggressive child population, is striking.

At follow-up, hyperactive and aggressive symptoms show a different course as well as different relationships to the environment. Many studies have suggested that the symptoms of inattention and hyperactive motor behavior tend to improve with increasing age. However, when aggressive behavior and self-esteem problems are present at an early age, they tend to remain or worsen over time. Moreover, the work of Loney and colleagues and Weiss and her colleagues has documented a significant relationship between aggressive behavior and adolescent outcome, and between parenting variables and adolescent outcome, while failing to find a relationship between hyperactive symptoms and adolescent outcome (Milich & Loney, 1979).

SOCIAL INFLUENCES AND DRUG EFFECTS

In a provocative review article Milich and Loney (1979) have hypothesized that the differential relationships of hyperactive and aggressive symptomatology to environmental variables and to adolescent outcome may explain some of the puzzles in the hyperkinesis treatment literature. One of these has to do with the fact that while stimulant medication results in short-term improvement in the primary symptoms of hyperkinesis, it has not been associated with long-term improvement.

According to Milich and Loney, since stimulant medication has its main effect on the primary symptoms, and since adolescent outcome is best predicted by secondary symptoms (and associated family interaction variables), medication treatment alone would not be expected to affect long-term outcome. These authors have hypothesized that although drug investigations are important, research effort might be better spent analyzing and treating aggression and environmental variables, if our goal is the long-term improvement of hyperkinetic children (Milich & Loney, 1979).

Implicit in this model is the assumption that the primary syndrome is time-limited and developmental in nature. Drugs may help in the short run, because they act directly upon the underlying mechanisms responsible for the major symptoms. But they do not act upon the social mechanisms that account for the secondary symptoms.

Any such model is necessarily an oversimplification. We believe that early family process, particularly events that lead to extremes of distress in the child, may leave a permanent mark upon the developing brain. The smooth evolution of progressively more refined and integrated brain structures may be severely disorganized by powerful social phenomena, such as child abuse, neglect, inconsistency, separation, or parental death. The high incidence of hyperkinesis among adopted and abused children probably reflects such influences, as well as genetic, traumatic, or perinatal influences on the brain. The biologically vulnerable child is in turn a powerful stimulus for maladaptive parenting, particularly in marginally functional social environments where the load of adverse influences upon development is high. Thus, it is difficult to disentangle the mutual biological and social influences, and distinction between primary and secondary influences is at best a useful heuristic device for asking questions.

RECIPROCAL PARENT-CHILD TRANSACTIONS

Most of the studies we have reviewed so far demonstrate a relationship between macroscopic parenting and family variables and child aggressive symptomatology. The fact that a relationship exists, however, does not necessarily imply a simple unidirectional influence in which poor parenting causes child symptomatology. In fact, there is a growing body of research showing that the social influences of parents and hyperkinetic children are reciprocal in nature with the behavior of each member of a parent-child dyad being influenced by the behavior of the other member. These studies suggest etiologic conclusions that poor parenting behavior causes child symptomatology are overly simplistic; the nature of the parent-child relationship is considerably more complex than originally believed.

Normal and Hyperactive Parent-Child Interactions

In the first of a series of studies addressed to these questions, Cunningham and Barkley (1979) observed 20 normal and 20 (unmedicated) hyperkinetic boys and their mothers interacting in free play and structured situations in which the mothers gave their children a series of tasks. Detailed behavioral observations were recorded by two highly trained observers using a coding system designed to capture the reciprocal, interdependent interactions of parent and child.

Significant differences between normal and hyperactive mother-child dyads emerged in both situations. In free play and task situations, mothers of hyperactives initiated significantly fewer social interactions with their children and responded to significantly fewer of their child's initiations to them. The most striking data in this regard showed that mothers of normal children responded positively to over 90% of their sons' interactions, whereas mothers of hyperactives ignored or responded negatively to 33% of their children's attempts to socialize.

In addition to these differences in social responsivity, mothers of hyperactives gave twice as many commands to their children in free play and task situations, and gave less overall praise and less contingent praise in task situations. The hyperkinetic children were significantly less compliant than normal children and displayed less sustained compliance than normals.

Bidirectional Parent-Child Influences

The previous study, showing that mothers of hyperkinetic children have a more coercive, controlling, and critical style, initiate fewer social interactions, and respond less to their children is consistent with those reviewed previously but does not clarify the bidirectional influence of parent and child behavior. Therefore, in their next study, Barkley and Cunningham (1979) utilized a triple-blind drug-placebo crossover design to study the effects of stimulant treatment on mother-child interaction in free play and task situations. That is, the children's behavior was modified using medication, but the mothers were not specifically asked to change their own behavior in any way.

In this study, marked changes were noted in the social behavior of both the children and their mothers. As might be expected, children increased their independent toy play, decreased their social initiations to their mothers, and increased their ability to initiate and sustain compliance to mother commands during drug treatment. Even more interesting were the effects of changes in the children's behavior on changes in the mothers' behavior. In free play, mothers increased their rate of positive response to child social initiations during the drug condition. In both free play and structured task they decreased their rate of commands and decreased their criticism of the child during the drug condition. Since mothers and observers were blind with respect to the drug and placebo conditions, changes in mother behavior can be attributed to changes in child behavior.

These studies by Barkley and Cunningham and similar studies by others (e.g., Humphries, Kinsbourne, & Swanson, 1978; Mash & Johnston, 1983) suggest that there is a high degree of behavioral reciprocity in the interactions of hyperkinetic children and their mothers. Mothers of unmedicated hyperkinetic children display a coercive, controlling, unresponsive parenting style. However, this style does not necessarily represent a static personality trait. Rather, coercive, controlling, critical parent behaviors are, at least in part, elicited by the hyperkinetic child's deficits in attention, impulse, and activity control. When these child problems are corrected, immediate decreases are seen in coercive parent behaviors.

Interestingly, however, decreases in coercive parent behavior do not correspond to increases to normal levels in positive parent behaviors in all situations. For example, if one looks closely at the Barkley studies, it can be seen that mothers of unmedicated hyperkinetic boys initiate fewer positive social interactions with their children than do mothers of normal boys in play situations; in addition, these mothers praise their children less than do mothers of normals (Cunningham & Barkley, 1979). However, even when the boys are treated with stimulant medications, there is no change in mother social initiations and no increase in the mother's rewards for child compliance in free play; neither is there an increase in the total amount of reward during a structured task (Barkley & Cunningham, 1979; Pollard, Ward, & Barkley, 1983).

These data lead one to speculate that negative parent behaviors and positive parent behaviors are not inversely related but represent two separate but correlated parenting dimensions. Negative parent behaviors seem to be directly influenced by the child's immediate behavior. Positive parent behaviors may be more influenced by the accumulation over time of interactive experiences between mother and child, and may be less responsive to momentary changes in the parent-child interaction. These speculations converge with those of Patterson (1983), who has suggested that families engaged in high rates of coercive, critical interaction over a period of time become more and more withdrawn and detached from one another and spend less and less pleasant time together.

In addition, studies of the family interactions of children with primary aggressive disorders have shown that parents of aggressive children can be differentiated from parents of normal children by the rate and topography of commands they deliver to their children. Not only do they deliver more commands, they deliver a higher rate of poorly formulated, unclear, nonspecific, or vague commands given in a threatening, angry, or nagging manner. Parents of aggressors have also been demonstrated to criticize their children at a higher rate and to display indifference or hostility toward their children. (For a review of this research see Wells & Forehand, 1981; Wells & Forehand, in press.)

These data suggest one possible model by which secondary symptoms of hyperkinetic syndrome develop. One might propose an interactive model in which the hyperkinetic child's impulsivity and short attention span evoke certain coercive, controlling parent behaviors that, in turn, promote and encourage child aggression via the mechanisms identified by Gerald Patterson (1983).

One difficulty with this model is that it does not explain why some hyperactive children develop secondary aggressive symptoms and others do not (Trites & Laprade, 1983). There may be individual differences in parenting styles that are evoked by hyperkinetic child behaviors, the identification of which has been obscured in group experimental designs reporting averaged data. In addition, while some parenting behaviors may be directly evoked in microscopic parent-child interactions, other parent behaviors may be more permanent and less dependent on the child's behavior. Likewise, after repeated evocation, some parents may make coercive, critical, punitive behaviors a permanent component of their parenting style, whereas others may be more able to resist the development of such a style.

Just as there may be typologies of hyperkinetic syndrome, there may also be typologies of parenting style that need to be identified. Such work is practically nonexistent. We can only echo Milich and Loney's (1979) call for more research identifying precisely the relationship between parenting and other social factors, and primary and secondary symptoms in hyperkinetic syndrome.

8

MULTIMODALITY TREATMENT

Hyperkinetic behavior is a complex phenomenon, having its origins in multiple influences from both biologic and social causes. Initial enthusiasm over the dramatic improvement in behavior from stimulant drugs led to unjustified optimism regarding the long-term therapeutic value of such treatments. At the same time, social and behavioral theorists, working in parallel and in isolation from medically oriented researchers, developed their own dogmas regarding the universality of behavioral therapies and often failed to recognize the fundamental biologic constraints upon adaptive learning in children who suffered from powerful derangements of impulse control, activity level, and attention. Only recently has systematic study of the various combinations of drug and behavioral treatments begun. Here we conclude our discussion of hyperkinesis with a review of the issues involved in the optimal treatment of these children and their families.

STIMULANT THERAPY AND BEHAVIOR THERAPY

Certainly the most ambitious, well-conducted, and influential studies of combined drug and behavior therapies have been conducted by Rachel Gittelman and colleagues. In 1976, and 1980, this group (Gittelman-Klein, Klein, Abikoff, Katz, Gloisten, & Kates, 1976; Gittelman et al., 1980) reported the results of a large-scale study designed to test the relative merits of stimulant medication versus behavior therapy, alone and combined. The experimental design employed in this study was a randomized but asymmetrical three-group design comparing MPH alone, MPH plus behavior therapy, and placebo plus behavior therapy.

The subjects were severely disruptive hyperactive children who received relatively high doses of MPH in the two drug conditions (up to 60 mg per day). Outcome measures consisted of factor scores from the Conners Teacher Rating Scale, global improvement ratings obtained from teachers, parents, and psychiatrists, and classroom behavioral data collected by independent trained observers who used a reliable and valid behavioral coding system. There were no measures of academic performance or achievement, social adjustment and status with peers, or home behavior (other than a global rating by parents). Furthermore, there was no follow-up assessment.

Results of this study revealed significant treatment effects from pre- to posttreatment for all three groups on the three relevant factors of the Conners Teacher Rating Scale (Conduct Disorder, Inattentive, Hyperactive). Significant effects from pre- to posttreatment were also found for two groups (MPH alone; MPH plus behavior therapy) on a composite measure of disruptive classroom behavior from the behavioral coding system. Teachers and psychiatrists rated 100% of the children in the combined-treatment group (MPH plus behavior therapy) as improved, whereas only a portion of the children in the other two groups (MPH alone; behavior therapy plus placebo) were rated as improved. Comparing treatments, the two drug-treated groups (MPH plus behavior therapy; MPH alone) were significantly more improved than the group receiving behavior therapy with placebo.

From a clinical perspective, the most important comparisons in the study were those comparing hyperactive children in each of the three treatment groups to normal classmate controls. At the end of treatment, there were no significant differences between hyperactive children who received the combined treatment (MPH plus behavior therapy) and normal children on any measures. In contrast, hyperactive children receiving MPH alone continued to be more disruptive and more solicitous of teacher attention than their normal comparisons. Hyperactive children who received behavior therapy plus placebo also continued to be more disruptive, more solicitous, and to display more minor motor movement than normal children. Thus, only a combined strategy of MPH plus behavior therapy completely normalized the behavior of hyperactive children. Neither strategy alone did so.

We have chosen to present this study in a fair amount of detail because, despite its elegance, it illustrates some of the methodological problems that continue to plague the treatment literature. In addition, this study serves as a focus for continued polemical arguments over what constitutes "the best therapy for hyperactive children." For example, in informal debates at national conventions, in discussions with some colleagues, and in our supervision sessions with psychiatry residents and interns, we have been disturbed to note the frequency with which the Gittelman et al. (1980) study is referenced to support statements such as "behavior therapy is ineffective with hyperactive children," "Stimulant therapy alone is the treatment of choice for hyperkinesis," and that it is "unnecessary to refer hyperactive children for adjunctive treatment." One trainee we supervised took great comfort from the Gittelman et al. (1980) study since (according to him) it meant that he did not "need to bother learning how to do behavioral and family therapy with my hyperactive patients." The generally excellent methodology of the study makes such conclusions appealing. But we believe that such conclusions are misguided (and certainly not intended by Gittelman and colleagues).

First, as pointed out by Ross and Ross (1982), the experimental design of the Gittelman et al. (1980) study was an asymmetrical, three-group design that failed to employ drug placebo only, behavior therapy only, attention-placebo, and no-treatment control groups. Commenting upon this design, Loney et al. (1979) note that "the change from baseline to follow-up in the group that received behavior therapy plus placebo cannot be confidently isolated as (1) a drug placebo effect, (2) a behavioral placebo effect, (3) a genuine behavioral therapy effect, or (4) some combination of the three. Because such an attribution cannot be made, it is possible that the behavioral treatment was merely ineffectively delivered and that the study therefore does not constitute a proper test of drug versus behavioral treatments" (1979, p. 135).

Gittelman et al. (1980) counter these comments on the quality of the behavior therapy in their study by pointing out that care was taken to hire individuals who had strong philosophical commitments to behavioral treatment. In addition, the magnitude of improvement obtained with behavioral treatment in the Gittelman study was similar to that obtained in other studies done at a university well known for research in behavior therapy (O'Leary, Pelham, Rosenbaum, & Price, 1976; Rosenbaum, O'Leary, & Jacob, 1975). We tend to agree with Gittelman on this point and are less concerned about it than we are about other methodological aspects of the study.

Two of the most important of these were the failure to employ multiple measures of outcome that assess the full range of symptomatology of the hyperkinetic impulse disorder (notably academic achievement and peer relationships), failure to evaluate the effects of high versus low doses of medication, and the failure to employ a follow-up phase. These are important omissions, for several reasons.

For reasons discussed in our presentation of drug therapy, a sizable literature suggests that improvements in academic performance and achievement do not occur with short- or long-term stimulant treatment alone (Barkley & Cunningham, 1978; Conrad, Dworkin, Shai, & Tobiessen, 1971; Gittelman-Klein & Klein, 1976; Hoffman et al., 1974; Riddle & Rapoport, 1976). However, there is suggestive evidence that behavioral treatment may result in improved academic performance (Ayllon, Layman, & Kandel, 1975; Pelham, Schnedler, Bologna, & Contreras, 1980; Wolraich, Drummond, Salomon, O'Brien, & Sivage, 1978). The fact that there were no measures of academic performance in Gittelman et al. (1980) precluded a conclusion that combined treatment most effectively treats the academic deficiencies of hyperactive children.

A similar point can be made about social skills and adjustment. We have good reason to be concerned about the social adjustment of hyperactive children. Both observational and sociometric data demonstrate that the peer relationships of these children are very seriously disturbed. Furthermore, early peer problems predict later maladjustment to a very significant extent as many follow-up studies have shown.

In the few studies assessing stimulant effects on peer relationships, treatment effects are not found (Pelham et al., in press). Whalen, Henker, Collins, Finck, & Dotemoto, 1979a), nor does stimulant treatment alone appear to be associated with long-term improvement in social behavior (Weiss et al., 1975). This has been especially disappointing since as hyperkinetic children grow older attention and activity problems improve, but their social adjustment does not improve.

In contrast, behavior therapy programs emphasizing social skills training (Bogart & Wells, 1985; Hinshaw, Henker, & Whalen, 1984; Pelham et al., in press) have demonstrated significant *short-term* improvements in social skills and peer relationships in hyperactive children on behavioral observations and sociometric measures. There are no follow-up studies of the long-term effects of behavioral treatment on peer relationships, so we do not know if combination treatments that include behavioral social skills training will improve the adult outcome of hyperkinetic children. The inclusion of sociometric and peer relationship measures and a follow-up evaluation in the Gittelman et al. (1980) study would have made the study much more clinically relevant, and might have resulted in a conclusion that behavior therapy with or without MPH results in improved social adjustment and peer relationships in hyperactive children.

The Gittelman et al. (1980) study can also serve to illustrate the importance of differentiating between clinical and statistical significance in evaluating questions of treatment efficacy. In this study, there were no statistically significant differences between groups of children receiving MPH alone versus MPH plus behavior therapy on teacher report or classroom observations. (Hence, the conclusions drawn by some that behavior therapy is unnecessary.)

However, teachers and psychiatrists rated 100% of the children who received the combined treatment as improved. Only 76% (teachers' ratings) and 81% (psychiatrists' ratings) receiving MPH alone were rated as improved, and 63% (teachers' ratings) and 58% (psychiatrists' ratings) receiving behavior therapy plus placebo were rated improved. Though the difference between 76% and 100% may not be statistically significant, it is certainly clinically significant for the children who were not viewed as improved by their teachers and psychiatrists on MPH alone.

Undoubtedly the most important point regarding clinical efficacy has to do with the normalizing effect of treatments. In the Gittelman et al. (1980) study only the group receiving the combined treatment (MPH plus behavior therapy) was indistinguishable from normal at the the end of the study on all measures. Children receiving MPH alone and behavior therapy plus placebo continued to display significant rates of abnormal behavior even though they had improved. Again, if one employs a standard of normal functioning, rather than statistically significant improvement, the combined treatment emerged as the best treatment.

In addition to these points, there are other reasons that nonpharmacological treatment modalities will continue to be employed. For example, relatively large doses of stimulants are usually needed to demonstrate significant and superior *behavioral* control of hyperactive children. [1] However, as noted earlier, there is evidence that high doses of stimulants may inhibit some cognitive performance and that much lower doses result in maximal cognitive effects (Peeke, Halliday, Callaway, Prael, & Reus, 1984; Sprague & Sleator, 1977). Thus, clinicians and teachers working with hyperkinetic children may have to sacrifice behavioral control in order to obtain the best effects on cognitive performance.

For these children, the combination of low-dose stimulant therapy with behavioral treatment for control of disruptive behavior may represent the best treatment. [2] In addition, concern about potentially adverse side effects related to high dose stimulant treatment (irritability, attenuation of growth, and weight gain) has prompted many clinicians to use smaller doses and to curtail the use of medication after school and on the weekends. Again, for these children who cannot tolerate the high doses of stimulants required for maximal behavioral control, combination treatments may be most clinically efficacious. Gittelman et al. (1980) did not include measures of cognitive function and academic performance, used high doses of MPH titrated to achieve behavioral control, and did not include measures of home behavior. Therefore, a conclusion that low-dose stimulant therapy combined with behavioral therapy represents optimal treatment was precluded.

The only other group outcome studies employing single versus combination conditions in the same design do not add much useful information to the debate because of serious methodological limitations in each study. For example, Pelham and Murphy (1985) have recently shown that data from one of the most frequently cited group studies of drug and behavioral treatment (Wolraich et al., 1978) are essentially uninterpretable due to serious design and statistical analysis problems.

Firestone, Kelly, Goodman, and Davey (1981) administered a behavior therapy program, parent training, which is designed to change children's behavior in the home setting, and then employed outcome measures relevant almost exclusively to the school setting. Changes in school behavior based on behavioral treatment in the home would not be expected (Forehand et al., 1979). Thus, neither of these group studies constitutes a reasonable experimental test of the hypothesis that combination treatments represent the most clinically efficacious approach for hyperactive children.

In contrast, recent studies employing single-subject experimental designs provide evidence that a treatment approach combining drug and behavioral interventions constitutes the most clinically efficacious approach. In the first of these, Pelham et al. (1980) studied the effects of a comprehensive sixteen-week behavioral program for eight hyperactive children. Three three-week MPH probes (before therapy and after three weeks and thirteen weeks of intervention), during which time placebo and low and high doses of MPH were administered, allowed for an evaluation of the effects of behavior therapy alone and behavior therapy combined with either low or high doses of stimulant treatment for each of the eight children.

Dependent measures consisted of classroom and clinic observations of disruptive and off-task behavior and teacher and parent ratings. Measures of academic performance were collected at pre- and posttreatment, but, unfortunately, not during medication probe phases. There were no measures of peer relationships and no follow-up assessment.

Results of this study showed that over the sixteen-week behavioral program, significant improvement was found from pre- to posttreatment in all the dependent measures, including academic performance. At both three weeks and thirteen weeks into the behavioral therapy, MPH significantly enhanced on-task behavior and teacher ratings of classroom behavior compared to behavior therapy plus placebo.

As a group, only when the eight children received behavioral intervention plus high-dose MPH did they reach a level of appropriate behavior similar to normal comparison children.[3] This is similar to the result obtained by Gittelman et al. (1980) on the superior effects of combined treatment in normalizing the behavior of hyperactive children. However, in contrast to Gittelman et al. (1980), the within-subjects design employed by Pelham et al. (1980) allowed for an analysis of the effects of the various treatments and their combination on individual children as well. These individual analyses revealed that two of the eight children were "normalized" with behavior therapy combined with low-dose therapy, one was normalized with behavior therapy alone, and one child never reached normal levels of function.

The Pelham et al. (1980) study essentially concurs with that of Gittelman in suggesting that behavior therapy is effective, but not maximally effective, for short-term treatment of the disruptive behavior of hyperactive children; that behavior therapy combined with medication is more effective than behavior therapy alone; and that only when a group of hyperactive children receive a combined treatment is their behavior normalized. As in Gittelman et al. (1980), no conclusions can be drawn regarding the long-term effects of these treatments, or the differential effects of these treatments on academic and social functioning.

The Pelham et al. (1980) study goes beyond the Gittelman study, however, in illustrating a point we have repeatedly made in previous publications (Conners & Wells, 1979; Wells, Conners, Imber, & Delamater, 1981), and one that is of great concern in clinical practice: the inability to generalize conclusions obtained in group studies to individual children. Conclusions drawn from studies employing group designs are based on statistical inferences made from averaged data and do not reflect individual variations within the sample. Individuals within a sample can and do vary with respect to their responses to treatments or combinations of treatments.

Thus, in Pelham et al. (1980), although the group as a whole showed its most significant improvement with behavior therapy combined with high-dose MPH, two of the children were normalized on behavior therapy combined with the low dose and one was normalized on behavior therapy alone. High doses of MPH for these three children represented unnecesssary overmedication. If clinicians are guided only by the results of group outcome studies, many such children will be unnecessarily overmedicated.

These points also serve to illustrate another important issue that we have repeatedly raised throughout this book: the extreme heterogeneity of what clinicians and researchers have referred to as "hyperkinesis," and the extent to which research efforts (particularly those employing group designs) have been hampered by the absence of a clear classification scheme.

Most group studies select subjects on the basis of a high hyperkinesis factor score leaving other dimensions of the syndrome (e.g., conduct problems, impulsivity, attentional problems) free to vary within the sample. Thus, children within a sample may be uniform with respect to hyperkinesis but may reflect different subtypes with respect to the presence or absence of other behavior dimensions. It is not surprising, therefore, that different children will respond to different treatments (or their combination) differently.

Recent studies by Wells et al. (1981) and Horn, Chatoor, and Conners (1983) demonstrate how single-subject designs can be used in a clinical setting to determine the most clinically efficacious approach for hyperactive children. These studies add further credence to our belief that combination treatments are more effective than stimulants alone or behavior therapy alone for highly disruptive, hyperactive children.

Both of these studies were conducted in child inpatient psychiatric settings. Results of Wells et al. (1981) are presented in Figure 8.1.

As seen in this figure, Dexedrine was essentially ineffective in controlling off-task and gross motor behavior of a hyperactive child, whereas MPH resulted in reduction in both behaviors compared to the preceding baseline and Dexedrine phases. However, the most significant improvement was obtained in Phase 5 when MPH was combined with a behavioral self-control program. When MPH was replaced by a placebo combined with self-control in Phase 6, off-task and gross motor behavior increased moderately. When MPH was again reinstated along with self-control in Phase 7 the relatively greater utility of the combined treatment was replicated.

Similarly, Horn et al. (1983) found that a combination of stimulant therapy and behavioral self-control training was more effective than either treatment alone in improving the classroom behavior of a hyperactive child. In addition, in this study neither Dexedrine nor self-control training improved academic performance. Only when Dexedrine was combined with reinforcement for academic responses was there improvement in this domain.

From a purely experimental perspective, single-subject designs have their own difficulties, although in our opinion the most frequently mentioned of these—poor external validity—is the least problematic. Critics usually suggest that because single-subject methodology employs small Ns, one cannot generalize their results to the larger population of hyperactive children. However, because of the heterogeneity of subject

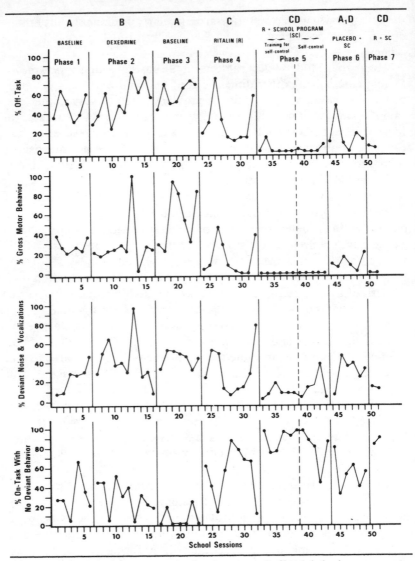

Figure 8.1. Percentage occurrence in the classroom of off-task behavior, gross motor behavior, deviant noise and vocalizations, and on-task behavior with no other deviant behavior recorded, measured across baseline, medication and placebo phases. From Wells, Conners, Imber, and Delameter (1981). Reprinted with permission of Pergamon Press.

samples in most group designs, they do not necessarily have greater external validity than single-subject designs.

The biggest problem with these designs is their inability to control order or sequence effects when several treatments are compared in the same individual. Only group designs provide true experimental control of order effects. Nevertheless, we have argued that if one assesses measurement reliability across all baseline and treatment phases, and employs a withdrawal design in which treatment is withdrawn and baseline levels of behavior are recovered before another treatment is implemented, single-subject experimental methodology can be used to compare differential effects of treatments in the clinical assessment process (Wells et al., 1981).

In summary, if we were to make a global generalization regarding the treatment of choice for hyperkinetic children, we would say that at a minimum, a combination of stimulant therapy and behavior therapy in the home and school represents the most clinically efficacious treatment. We base this statement on the small number of studies in the literature, with minimally adequate experimental methodology, that have compared combination treatments to univariate treatment. However, this literature is not extensive, and each study has limitations that prevent a sweeping definitive conclusion at present. We also base our judgment regarding the effectiveness of combination treatments on certain (empirically based) theoretical assumptions we have made throughout this book regarding the nature of hyperkinesis. At a global level of analysis, we have presumed that "hyperkinesis" is an umbrella term that encompasses a constellation of symptoms from dimensions of impulsivity, attention, and other perceptual/cognitive processes, activity, and conduct, each of which may have primary biologic and environmental contributions to its etiology.

To the extent that stimulant therapy and behavior therapy have a differential impact on these dimensions, it is likely that combination treatment will most effectively treat children who display extreme symptoms or the full array of symptoms. For example, evidence suggests that stimulants have an immediate but short-lived effect on attention and activity (Solanto & Conners, 1982), while behavior therapy has its primary impact on aggressive behavior (Abikoff & Gittelman, 1984). Nevertheless, it is clear that stimulants alone also improve conduct problems and that behavior therapy alone results in some improvement in attention and activity problems (Abikoff & Gittelman, 1984; Gittelman et al., 1980). To the extent that neither treatment alone results in maximal improvement in each dimension, combining them may allow their additive effects to more closely approximate fully normalizing treatment. This, in fact, seems to have been demonstrated in studies showing that normalization of function only occurs with combination treatment (Gittelman et al., 1980; Pelham et al., 1980).

At the macroscopic level of analysis we have presumed that hyperkinesis constitutes a constellation of symptoms. However, we have also presumed that individual children may vary in the extent and degree to which dysfunction in each dimension is present, and the extent to which each dimension is driven by biological and environmental influences. We have speculated that subtypes representing different clusters of the fundamental dimensions may be identified in clinic and normal population. As we become more sophisticated in defining subtypes of the hyperkinetic impulse disorder, we may find that some subtypes are, in fact, maximally treated with stimulant therapy or behavior therapy alone and that other subtypes require combination treatments for maximal and completely normalizing effects. As yet no studies have looked at the interaction between subtypes and treatment outcome for stimulant therapy, behavior therapy, and their combination in the same experimental design.

Just as the term "hyperkinetic impulse disorder" is a global concept encompassing different combinations of symptom patterns, so too are the terms "behavior therapy" and "stimulant treatment" global labels as we have used them in this chapter. For example, there are three stimulant medications in common usage with children and each is administered at varying dosage levels depending upon the clinical practices of individual physicians. Likewise, "behavior therapy" encompasses many technologies, from parent training to operant reinforcement of academic responses. Given the diversity of subject and treatment characteristics in this field, the question, "What is the treatment of choice for hyperactive children?" is too global in scope for our present state of knowledge. Rather, the question, "Which level of medication, and/or which set of behavior therapy procedures is most helpful for which subtypes of hyperkinetic child on which symptoms and in which situations?" though more semantically awkward, is also more to the point. We believe that the field needs many more individual single-subject and small N studies in which the descriptive characteristics of the particular children being studied are very carefully spelled out, the nature of the behavior therapy techniques is carefully documented, the nature of the situation or context in which treatment is delivered is carefully described, and the outcome measures are carefully planned.

OTHER THERAPY MODALITIES

Although stimulant therapy and behavior therapy are by far the most widely researched interventions for hyperkinesis, there is reason to believe that other therapy modalities may also add to the effects of these two treatments. Addition of these modalities may be especially important for those children who do not experience maximal treatment effects from stimulants and behavior therapy (recall the one child in Pelham et al. (1980) who had not reached normal function with the combination treatment). In addition, some children may not tolerate stimulant therapy because of side effects, and some families and teachers may not cooperate with behavioral or stimulant treatment. For these children other therapy modalities are needed.

Individual Psychotherapy

Most contemporary authorities have conceptualized the primary symptoms of the hyperkinetic impulse disorder as arising from a complex interplay of the temperamental and / or biological condition of the organism with the parenting and school environments. This conceptual model, along with the results of a few studies showing no effects of traditional treatments on hyperkinetic children (Eisenberg et al., 1961), has led to a belief that individual psychotherapy has very little to offer the hyperkinetic child. We tend to agree that traditional psychotherapy is not particularly useful for the primary symptoms of the syndrome. However, we also agree with a group of investigators who have argued that psychotherapy may be a useful adjunct to stimulant and behavioral therapy, particularly for the secondary symptoms or sequelae of the syndrome such as poor self-esteem, anxiety, and depression (Cantwell, 1979; Satterfield, Cantwell, & Satterfield, 1979). However, psychotherapy for these conditions would not be expected to affect the child's hyperkinesis. Therefore, when individual psychotherapy is provided to hyperkinetic children, it should be provided as an adjunct, not a substitute, to stimulant and / or behavioral treatment.

Multimodality Psychotherapy

Over the past five years, Satterfield and his colleagues (Satterfield et al., 1979; Satterfield, Satterfield, & Cantwell, 1980; 1981) have conducted a large-scale study evaluating the effects of a so-called total push treatment program involving several therapeutic modalities (drug therapy, individual therapy, and educational therapy for the child, and parent training, couples, group and family therapy for the parents). Treatment planning was individualized so that each family received some or all of these modalities. At the three-year evaluation, these investigators have found unexpectedly good outcome on behavioral and academic measures for hyperactive children who remained in treatment for the entire three years, but not for those who dropped out after one year.

The results for the three-year intensive treatment group also compare favorably to other follow-up studies using less intensive or no treatment, providing suggestive evidence that total push drug, psychotherapeutic, and behavioral therapy (parent training) improves the long-term outcome for these children. Unfortunately, in the absence of certain methodological standards, the results are only suggestive, and in some ways the study raises more questions than it answers.

For example, we do not know if all the modalities are necessary or if only a subset are required for children to reach an asymptote of improvement. Likewise, families who stay in treatment for three years may be a very different sample than those who drop out, and improvement for the three-year children may be related more to family characteristics than to the effects of treatment. Finally, families who are seen in treatment weekly for three years may be more likely to comply with medication than those who drop out; beneficial effects at three years may be due primarily to the greater compliance with medication than for groups who have no contact with a therapist.

In spite of interpretive problems that arise from this series of studies, it does suggest that there is something about being involved in intensive treatment for a long period (at least three years) that may improve the outcome for hyperactive children; and for families who can afford it, intensive multimodality treatment might be recommended on that basis. However, because many families will not or cannot participate in this type of intensive treatment, component analyses of multimodality treatment should be undertaken to determine if similar effects can be obtained with less intensive and expensive treatment.

Cognitive Therapy

Since the publication of Meichenbaum and Goodwin's (1971) study of a cognitive self-instructional training program for impulsive children there has been increasing interest in the efficacy of cognitive therapies for the hyperkinetic impulse disorder. This approach has been most strongly advocated by Virginia Douglas (1975, 1980) and represents a logical outgrowth of her primary research interest in the cognitive/perceptual characteristics of hyperactive children.

Douglas has advocated cognitive therapy on the basis of certain theoretical assumptions she made regarding the fundamental mechanisms of hyperkinesis. She has stated, "Most of the disabilities that define the hyperactive syndrome can be traced to deficits in three related processes. These include mechanisms governing: (a) the investment of attention and effort; (b) the inhibition of impulsive responding; and (c) the modulation of arousal level to meet situational or task demands" (1980, p. 284). Douglas has further argued that if treatment is to be effective it must be directed toward these defective processes, and has stated her belief that cognitive therapy offers the most promise in this regard.

Unfortunately, while this theoretical model has a certain appeal, the existing data do not strongly support cognitive therapy alone as a viable alternative to stimulant therapy and/or behavior therapy for hyperkinetic syndrome (Abikoff & Gittelman, 1983), although it may be a useful adjunct for promoting cognitive performance (Douglas, Parry, Marton, & Gaston, 1976). Even so, some studies have reported no effects of cognitive therapy (Eastman & Rasbury, 1981; Friedling & O'Leary, 1979), and those that do report significant treatment effects also place heavy emphasis on overt reinforcement and contingency management as part of the cognitive training (Bornstein & Quevillon, 1976; Douglas et al., 1976). Thus, it is impossible to tease apart the unique contribution of cognitive therapy in these studies since the reinforcement procedures alone may be responsible for the effects.

Our basis for believing that cognitive therapy has only limited usefulness for hyperactive children stems from its failure to effect the full range of symptomatology of the hyperkinetic syndrome. For example, Douglas et al. (1976) found that after a three-month treatment program, significant improvement compared to no treatment was found on error and time scores on the Matching Familiar Figures Test (a measure of cognitive impulsivity), aggressive and realistic coping responses on a story completion test and the time measure on the Bender-Gestalt (errors on the Bender did not improve). Unfortunately, effects on cognitive performance did not seem to mediate improvement in reading and arithmetic achievement or classroom behavior. No significant effects compared to no treatment were found on three of four subtests of the Durrell Analysis of Reading Difficulty, on the WRAT Arithmetic Scale, or on the Conners Teacher Rating Scale.

Similarly, Meichenbaum and Goodman (1971) found that while cognitive training improved certain cognitive performance measures (Picture Arrangement Subtest of the WISC; latency score on the MFF; errors on the Porteus Maze Test), no effects of treatment were found on the children's classroom behavior or on teacher ratings.

In addition to these somewhat discouraging results, Abikoff and Gittelman (1983) have recently reported preliminary results from their large-scale group outcome study assessing the comparative efficacy of stimulant medication alone versus stimulant medication plus cognitive therapy. In this study cognitive training occurred for sixteen weeks, even longer than that delivered by Douglas et al. (1976). Preliminary analyses of 39 children indicated no group differences on 65 out of 67 teacher and parent measures of behavior, and no differences on the WRAT subtests, the Gray Oral Reading Test or the Stanford Achievement Test, all measures of academic achievement.

The only measures on which children receiving cognitive therapy plus medication did better than those receiving medication alone was the Paired Associates Learning Test. Thus, the interim results from this study found no statistically significant benefit from adding cognitive therapy to medication treatment compared to medication alone. However, our comments in an earlier section regarding the importance of differentiating between statistical and clinical significance also pertain here. In addition, analyses of data from individual children may show that some did benefit from the addition of cognitive therapy. Therefore, final judgment regarding the clinical usefulness of cognitive therapy combined with stimulants must await the final report from these authors.

At the present time, we can only conclude that if cognitive therapy has any benefits for the hyperactive child, those benefits appear to be very limited when compared to the effects obtained with stimulant therapy and behavior therapy. It was initially hoped that cognitive therapy would improve the academic achievement of hyperactive children. However, neither of the two longer trials of cognitive therapy has shown any appreciable improvements in academic achievement compared to no treatment (Douglas et al., 1976) or to stimulant treatment alone (Abikoff & Gittelman, 1983).

The only conclusion that can be drawn at present is that cognitive therapy may help certain cognitive and problem-solving deficiencies of hyperactive children; unfortunately, these improvements do not appear to mediate improvement in the academic or behavioral aspects of the syndrome.

Relaxation Therapy

Interest in the use of relaxation training as an adjunctive treatment for hyperkinesis has grown since the first use of this approach by Braud, Lupin, and Braud (1975). These and other authors have theorized that muscular tension and heightened neurophysiological arousal contribute to and exacerbate the symptoms of hyperactivity, and that relaxation training can be useful in teaching the child to reduce tension and arousal. At least one well-designed study has demonstrated that significant differences in EMG muscle tension levels do exist between hyperactive and nonhyperactive subjects prior to treatment.

In the first case study of this treatment approach, Braud et al. (1975) employed EMG biofeedback to teach relaxation skills to a 6½-year-old extremely hyperactive boy. This child learned to decrease muscle tension levels to a very significant extent both within and across his eleven treatment sessions. Activity, tension, and emotionality ratings taken at each training session declined consistently across the sessions. Parent and teacher global reports indicated general behavioral improvement as well as significant improvement in the hours after the training sessions. Improvements were also noted on psychological and achievement testing.

The results of this uncontrolled case study, while inconclusive, have encouraged other investigators to evalute the effectiveness of relaxation therapy. Some of the studies have shown that relaxation training is associated with improvements in hyperactive children's's test performance, as well as certain primary symptoms of hyperkinetic syndrome (Braud, 1978; Denkowski, Denkowski, & Omizo, 1983; Dunn & Howell, 1982; Omizo & Michael, 1982). However, one of the best-designed studies has shown that relaxation training has its most significant effect on the secondary symptoms of the syndrome (e.g., emotionality, irritability, aggression; see Braud, 1978).

In this important study, fifteen hyperkinetic children were randomly assigned to three experimental groups: biofeedback-induced relaxation, progressive relaxation training, and hyperactive control. After twelve treatment sessions, significant improvements were seen in muscular tension, on parent ratings, and on psychological test performance for both treatment groups compared to the control group. The greatest behavioral improvement was seen in emotionality/aggression, though other primary behavioral symptoms also improved.

Results such as these suggest that relaxation therapies show good potential as adjunctive treatments for hyperkinetic children. They contribute to improvements in both primary and secondary symptoms as well as psychological test performance. They seem particularly useful in treatment of secondary symptoms such as emotional lability, low self-esteem, and explosive-aggressive behavior. As indicated earlier, tonic efferent inflow of stimulation from the periphery may be actually enhanced by relaxation.

CONCLUSIONS

The data we have reviewed in this chapter lead us to conclude that for highly disruptive hyperactive children, a multimodal treatment approach including, at a minimum, stimulant therapy and behavior therapy will be necessary to treat the full range of symptoms of the disorder. In addition, for children experiencing other sequelae of the disorder, other individual, group, and family psychotherapeutic modalities may be useful. When stimulant medication is used with school-aged children the dose should be adjusted to achieve the best effects on academic and cognitive performance. The use of academic performance as the target of stimulant dosage titration may or may not result in maximal behavioral control. For those children who continue to experience behavioral problems with the lower doses that are typically needed to attain the best cognitive effects, behavior therapy procedures should be implemented (see O'Leary & O'Leary, 1977). In addition, behavioral parent training (see Forehand & McMahon, 1981) can be used in treatment of home problems for children who do not receive stimulant medication in the afternoons or on weekends, or for those who do not achieve maximal behavioral control with stimulants alone.

Because it appears that many children will not show improvements in their social and peer relationships with stimulant and standard behavior therapy, we believe that social skills training will increasingly be employed with hyperactive children. Research in this area is just beginning to occur; however, the recent study by Hinshaw et al. (1984) is exemplary of such an approach. Group psychotherapy emphasizing social skills modeling and roleplaying procedures may be very useful with hyperactive children.

While multimodal treatment may be necessary for highly disruptive hyperactive children who display the full range of symptomatology, more circumscribed treatment may be sufficient for pure subtypes. For example, in an important study of the interrelationship of dimensions of psychopathology in a large sample of school children (n = 14,083) Trites and Laprade (1983) found that 2.0% of the sample were clinically hyperactive but displayed no conduct problems, while 3.7% displayed clinical hyperkinesis and conduct problems. We may find that single modality treatments (e.g., stimulants alone) will be sufficient for the former subgroup (pure hyperactives) whereas multimodality treatment will more likely be necessary for the combined hyperactive/conduct problems group. Because of their greater maladjustment, it is precisely these children, displaying the combination of hyperactive and aggressive symptomatology, who are most likely to be referred to clinics for treatment. Therefore, clinicians must increasingly become skilled in the application of multimodality treatment approaches and the use of single-case experimental designs in the clinical setting.

NOTES

1. In Gittelman et al. (1980) the average dose was 38.2 mg/day with a maximum of 60 mg/day.

2. There is now evidence that when multimodality treatment is provided, lower doses of stimulants can be used. For example, Satterfield et al. (1980) have found that by combining stimulant therapy with an individualized, multimodality treatment an average of 27.5 mg/day of MPH was needed for maximal behavioral control. In contrast, Gittelman et al. (1980) employed an average of 38 mg/day to obtain maximal behavioral control when medication was the only treatment. Interestingly, Satterfield et al. (1980) found improvement in academic achievement after two years of multimodality treatment, in contrast to other studies employing higher doses of stimulants and finding no improvement (e.g., Riddle and Rapoport, 1976).

3. Unfortunately, since measures of academic performance were obtained only at pre- and posttreatment, and not during the placebo and MPH probes, it was not possible to evaluate the effects of low versus high doses on academic measures.

APPENDIX

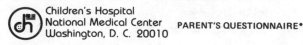

Children's Hospital
National Medical Center
Washington, D. C. 20010   **PARENT'S QUESTIONNAIRE***

OFFICE USE
Patient No.
Study No.

Name of Child _____   Date _____

Your Name _____ Relationship _____

I. Instructions: Listed below are items concerning children's behavior or the problems they sometimes have. Read each item carefully and decide how much you think your child has been bothered by this problem <u>during the past month</u> — NOT AT ALL, JUST A LITTLE, PRETTY MUCH, or VERY MUCH

Indicate your choice by placing a check mark (√) in the appropriate column to the right of each item.

ANSWER ALL ITEMS.

Observation	Not at all	Just a little	Pretty much	Very much
PROBLEMS OF EATING				
1. Picky and finicky				
2. Will not eat enough				
3. Overweight				
PROBLEMS OF SLEEP				
4. Restless				
5. Nightmares				
6. Awakens at night				
7. Cannot fall asleep				
FEAR AND WORRIES				
8. Afraid of new situations				
9. Afraid of people				
10. Afraid of being alone				
11. Worries about illness and death				
MUSCULAR TENSION				
12. Gets stiff and rigid				
13. Twitches, jerks, etc.				
14. Shakes				
SPEECH PROBLEMS				
15. Stuttering				
16. Hard to understand				
WETTING				
17. Bed wetting				
18. Runs to bathroom constantly				
BOWEL PROBLEMS				
19. Soiling self				
20. Holds back bowel movements				

*Questionnaire design by C. Keith Conners, Ph.D.

Form 4

142

2

ANSWER ALL ITEMS

Observation	Not at all	Just a little	Pretty much	Very much
COMPLAINS OF FOLLOWING SYMPTOMS EVEN THOUGH DOCTOR CAN FIND NOTHING WRONG				
21. Headaches				
22. Stomach aches				
23. Vomiting				
24. Aches and pains				
25. Loose bowels				
PROBLEMS OF SUCKING, CHEWING or PICKING				
26. Sucks thumb				
27. Bites or picks nails				
28. Chews on clothes, blankets, or others				
29. Picks at things such as hair, clothing, etc.				
CHILDISH OR IMMATURE				
30. Does not act his age				
31. Cries easily				
32. Wants help doing things he should do alone				
33. Clings to parents or other adults				
34. Baby talk				
TROUBLE WITH FEELINGS				
35. Keeps anger to himself				
36. Lets himself get pushed around by other children				
37. Unhappy				
38. Carries a chip on his shoulder				
OVER-ASSERTS HIMSELF				
39. Bullying				
40. Bragging and boasting				
41. Sassy to grown-ups				
PROBLEMS MAKING FRIENDS				
42. Shy				
43. Afraid they do not like him				
44. Feelings easily hurt				
45. Has no friends				
PROBLEMS WITH BROTHERS AND SISTERS				
46. Feels cheated				
47. Mean				
48. Fights constantly				

3

ANSWER ALL ITEMS

Observation	Not at all	Just a little	Pretty much	Very much
PROBLEMS KEEPING FRIENDS				
49. Disturbs other children				
50. Wants to run things				
51. Picks on other children				
RESTLESS				
52. Restless or over active				
53. Excitable, impulsive				
54. Fails to finish things he starts—short attention span				
TEMPER				
55. Temper outbursts, explosive and unpredictable behavior				
56. Throws himself around				
57. Throws and breaks things				
58. Pouts and sulks				
SEX				
59. Plays with own sex organs				
60. Involved in sex play with others				
61. Modest about his body				
PROBLEMS IN SCHOOL				
62. Is not learning				
63. Does not like to go to school				
64. Is afraid to go to school				
65. Daydreams				
66. Truancy				
67. Will not obey school rules				
LYING				
68. Denies having done wrong				
69. Blames others for his mistakes				
70. Tells stories which did not happen				
STEALING				
71. From parents				
72. At school				
73. From stores and other places				
FIRE-SETTING				
74. Sets fires				
TROUBLE WITH POLICE				
75. Gets into trouble with police				
Why?				

4

ANSWER ALL ITEMS

Observation	Not at all	Just a little	Pretty much	Very much
PERFECTIONISM				
76. Everything must be just so				
77. Things must be done same way every time				
78. Sets goals too high				
ADDITIONAL PROBLEMS				
79. Inattentive, easily distracted				
80. Constantly fidgeting				
81. Cannot be left alone.				
82. Always climbing				
83. A very early riser				
84. Will run around between mouthfuls at meals				
85. Demands must be met immediately—easily frustrated				
86. Cannot stand too much excitement.				
87. Laces and zippers are always open				
88. Cries often and easily				
89. Unable to stop a repetitive activity				
90. Acts as if driven by a motor.				
91. Mood changes quickly and drastically				
92. Poorly aware of surroundings or time of day				
93. Still cannot tie his shoelaces				

II. Please add any other problems you have with your child.

_____

_____

_____

_____

_____

_____

_____

III. How serious a problem do you think your child has at this time?

(   ) No Problem   (   ) Minor Problem   (   ) Serious Problem

IV. Indicate the items you are most concerned about or those you think are the most important problems your child has by placing a circle around the number (1-93) of those items.

REFERENCES

Abikoff, H., & Gittelman, R. (1983). *Cognitive training and stimulant medication in hyperactive children: Summary of results.* Unpublished manuscript.

Abikoff, H., & Gittelman, R. (1984). Does behavior therapy normalize the classroom behavior of hyperactive children? *Archives of General Psychiatry, 41,* 449-454.

Abikoff, H., Gittelman, R., & Klein, D. F. (1980). Classroom observation code for hyperactive children: A replication of validity. *Journal of Clinical and Consulting Psychology, 48,* 555-565.

Abikoff, H., Gittelman-Klein, R., & Klein, D. F. (1977). Validation of a classroom observation code for hyperactive children. *Journal of Consulting and Clincial Psychology, 45,* 772-783.

American Psychiatric Association. (1968). *Diagnostic and statistical manual of mental disorders* (2nd ed.). Washington, DC: Author.

American Psychiatric Association. (1980). *Diagnostic and statistical manual of mental disorders* (3rd ed.). Washington, DC: Author.

August, G. J., Stewart, M. A., & Holmes, C. S. (1983). A four-year follow-up of hyperactive boys with and without conduct disorder. *British Journal of Psychiatry, 143,* 192-198.

Ayllon, T., Layman, D., & Kandel, H. J. (1975). A behavioral-educational alternative to control of hyperactive children. *Journal of Applied Behavior Analysis, 8,* 137-146.

Barkley, R. A. (1976). Predicting the response of hyperkinetic children to stimulant drugs: A review. *Journal of Abnormal Child Psychology, 4,* 327-348.

Barkley, R. A. (1977). The effects of methylphenidate on various types of activity level and attention in hyperkinetic children. *Journal of Abnormal Child Psychology, 5,* 351-369.

Barkley, R. A. (1979). Stimulant drugs in the classroom. *School Psychology Digest, 8,* 412-425.

Barkley, R. A. (1981). *Hyperactive children: A handbook for diagnosis and treatment.* New York: Guilford.

Barkley, R. A., & Cunningham, C. E. (1978). Do stimulant drugs improve the academic performance of hyperkinetic children? A review of outcome studies. *Clinical Pediatrics, 17,* 85-92.

Barkley, R. A., & Cunningham, C. E. (1979). The effects of methylphenidate on the mother-child interactions of hyperactive children. *Archives of General Psychiatry, 36,* 201-208.

Barkley, R. A., & Jackson, T. L. (1977). Hyperkinesis, autonomic nervous system activity, and stimulant drug effects. *Journal of Child Psychology and Psychiatry, 18,* 347-357.

Barkley, R. A., & Ullman, D. G. (1975). A comparison of objective measures of activity and distractability in hyperactive and nonhyperactive children. *Journal of Abnormal Child Psychology, 3,* 231-244.

Beaumont, J. G. (1983). *Introduction to neuropsychology.* New York: Guilford.

Bell, R. Q. (1968). Adaptation of small wrist watches for mechanical recording of activity in infants and children. *Journal of Experimental Child Psychology, 6,* 302-305.

Birch, H. G. (1964). *Brain damage in children: The biological and social aspects.* Baltimore: Williams & Wilkins.

Bloomingdale, L. M., Davies, R. K., & Gold, M. S. (1984). Some possible neurological substrates in attention deficit disorder. In L. M. Bloomingdale (Ed.), *Attention deficit disorder: Diagnostic, cognitive and therapeutic understanding.* New York: Spectrum.

Blouin, A. G., Conners, C. K., & Seidel, W. T. (unpublished). *The independence of hyperactivity from conduct disorder: Methodological considerations.*

Bogart, C., & Wells, K. C. (1985). *Effects of social skills training with hyperactive children on the psychiatric inpatient unit.* Unpublished manuscript.

Bornstein, P. H., & Quevillon, R. P. (1976). The effects of a self-instructional package on overactive preschool boys. *Journal of Applied Behavior Analysis, 9,* 179-188.

Bradley, C. (1937). The behavior of children receiving benzedrine. *American Journal of Psychiatry, 94,* 577-585.

Bradley, C. (1950). Benzedrine and dexedrine in the treatment of children's behavior disorders. *Pediatrics, 5,* 24-36.

Braud, L. W. (1978). The effects of frontal EMG biofeedback and progressive relaxation upon hyperactivity and its behavioral concomitants. *Biofeedback and Self-Regulation, 3,* 69-88.

Braud, L. W., Lupin, M. N., & Braud, W. G. (1975). The use of electromyographic biofeedback in the control of hyperactivity. *Journal of Learning Disabilities, 8,* 21-26.

Bremner, J. G. (1982). Object localization in infancy. In M. Potegal (Ed.), *Spatial abilities: Development and physiological foundations.* New York: Academic Press.

Brobeck, J. R. (1979). *Best and Taylor's physiological basis of medical practice* (10th ed.). Baltimore: Williams & Wilkins.

Buss, A. H., & Plomin, R. (1975). *A temperament theory of personality development.* New York: Wiley.

Buss, A. H., Plomin, R., & Willerman, L. (1973). The inheritance of temperaments. *Journal of Personality, 41,* 513-524.

Buss, D. M., Block, J. H., & Block J. (1980). Preschool activity level: Personality correlates and developmental implications. *Child Development, 51,* 401-408.

Callaway, E., & Halliday, R. (1982). The effect of attentional effort on visual evoked potential N1 latency. *Psychiatry Research, 7,* 299-308.

Callaway, E., Halliday, R., & Naylor, H. (1983). Hyperactive children's event-related potentials fail to support under-arousal and maturational-lag theories. *Archives of General Psychiatry, 40,* 1243-1248.

Campbell, S. (1975). Mother-child interaction: A comparison of hyperactive, learning disabled, and normal boys. *Developmental Psychology, 45,* 51-57.

Cantwell, D. P. (1972). Psychiatric illness in the families of hyperactive children. *Archives of General Psychiatry, 27,* 414-417.

Cantwell, D. P. (1975). Clinical picture, epidemiology and classifications of the hyperactive child syndrome. In D. P. Cantwell (Ed.), *The hyperactive child: Diagnosis, management, current research.* New York: Spectrum.

Cantwell, D. P. (1979). The "hyperactive" child. *Hospital Practice, 14,* 65-73.

Cantwell, D. P. (1983). Diagnostic validity of the hyperactive child (attention deficit disorder with hyperactivity) syndrome. *Psychiatric Developments, 3,* 277-300.

Casey, P. (1977). The hyperactive child: Review and suggested management. *Texas Medicine, 73,* 68-75.

Cattell, R. B. (1957). *Handbook for the IPAT Anxiety Scale (Self Analysis Form).* Champaign, Il: IPAT.

Clements, S. D. (1966). *Task force one: Minimal brain dysfunction in children.* Washington, DC: National Institute of Neurological Diseases and Blindness, Monograph No. 3, DHEW.

Clyde, D. J. (1963). *Manual for the Clyde Mood Scale.* Miami: University of Miami Press.

Cohen, N. J., & Douglas, V. I. (1972). Characteristics of the orienting response in hyperactive and normal children. *Psychophysiology, 9,* 238-245.

Colburn, T., Smith, B. M., & Guarini, J. (1976). An ambulatory activity monitor with solid-state memory. *ISA Transactions, 15,* 149-154.

Conners, C. K. (1970). Symptom patterns in hyperkinetic, neurotic, and normal children. *Child Development, 41,* 667-682.

Conners, C. K. (1971). The effect of stimulant drugs on human figure drawings in children with minimal brain dysfunction. *Psychopharmacologia, 19,* 329-333.

Conners, C. K. (1972). Stimulant drugs and cortical evoked responses in learning and behavior disorders in children. In W. L. Smith (Ed.), *Drugs, development and cerebral function.* Springfield, Il: Charles C Thomas.

Conners, C. K. (1973). Rating scales. In *Psychopharmacology Bulletin: Special issue on pharmacotherapy of children.* Washington, DC: NIMH, Government Printing Office.

Conners, C. K. (1975a). Minimal brain dysfunction and psychopathology in children. In A. Davids (Ed.), *Child personality and psychopathology: Current topics.* New York: Wiley.

Conners, C. K. (1975b). Psychological assessment of children with minimal brain dysfunction. *Annals of the New York Academy of Sciences, 205,* 283-302.

Conners, C. K., & Applebee, A. (unpublished). *Methods for delineating subtypes of minimal brain dysfunction.*

Conners, C. K., & Eisenberg, L. (1963). The effects of methylphenidate on symptomatology and learning in disturbed children. *American Journal of Psychiatry, 120,* 458-463.

Conners, C. K., Eisenberg, L., & Sharpe, L. (1964). Effects of methylphenidate (Ritalin) on paired associate learning and Porteus Maze performance in emotionally disturbed children. *Journal of Consulting Psychology, 28,* 14-22.

Conners, C. K., & Greenfeld, D. (1966). Habituation of motor startle in anxious and restless children. *Journal of Child Psychology and Psychiatry, 7,* 125-132.

Conners, C. K., & Rothschild, G. H. (1968). Drugs and learning in children. In J. Hellmuth (Ed.), *Learning disorders* (Vol. 3). Seattle: Special Child Publications.

Conners, C. K., & Solanto, M. V. (1984). The psychophysiology of stimulant drug response in hyperkinetic children. In L. M. Bloomingdale (Ed.), *Attention deficit disorder: Diagnostic, cognitive, and therapeutic understanding.* New York: Spectrum.

Conners, C. K., & Taylor, E. (1980). Pemoline, methylphenidate, and placebo in children with minimal brain dysfunction. *Archives of General Psychiatry, 37,* 922-930.

Conners, C. K., & Wells, K. C. (1979). Method and theory for psychopharmacology with children. In R. L. Trites (Ed.), *Hyperactivity in children: Etiology, measurement, and treatment indications.* Baltimore: University Park Press.

Conners, C. K., & Werry, J. S. (1979). Pharmacotherapy. In H. C. Quay & J. S. Werry (Eds.), *Psychopathological disorders of childhood* (2nd ed.). New York: Wiley.

Conners, C. K., Taylor, E., Meo, G., Kurtz, M. A., & Fournier, M. (1972). Magnesium pemoline and dextroamphetamine: A controlled study in children with minimal brain dysfunction. *Psychopharmacologia, 26,* 321-336.

Conrad, W. G., Dworkin, E. S., Shai, A., & Tobiessen, J. E. (1971). Effects of amphetamine therapy and prescriptive tutoring on the behavior and achievement of lower-class hyperactive children. *Journal of Learning Disabilities, 4,* 509-517.

Crider, A., & Lunn, R. (1971). Electrodermal lability as a personality dimension. *Journal of Experimental Research in Personality, 5,* 145-150.

Cromwell, R., Baumeister, A., & Hawkins, W. (1963). Research in activity level. In N. Ellis (Ed.), *Handbook of mental deficiency.* New York: McGraw-Hill.

Cunningham, C. E., & Barkley, R. A. (1979). The interactions of normal and hyperactive children with their mothers in free play and structured tasks. *Child Development, 50,* 217-224.

Cytryn, L., Gilbert, A., & Eisenberg, L. (1960). The effectiveness of tranquilizing drugs plus supportive psychotherapy in treating behavior disorders of children: A double-blind study. *American Journal of Orthopsychiatry, 30,* 113-129.

Dainer, K. B., Klorman, R., Salzman, L. F., Hess, D. W., Davidson, P. W., & Michael, R. L. (1981). Learning-disordered children's evoked potentials during sustained attention. *Journal of Abnormal Child Psychology, 9,* 79-94.

Damasio, A. R., & Hoesen, G.W.V. (1983). Emotional disturbances associated with focal lesions of the limbic frontal lobe. In K. M. Heilman & P. Satz (Eds.), *Neuropsychology of human emotion.* New York: Guilford.

Davis, G. D. (1957). Effects of central exciting and depressant drugs on locomotor activity in the monkey. *American Journal of Physiology, 188,* 619-623.

Davis, R. C. (1948). Motor effects of strong auditory stimuli. *Journal of Experimental Psychology, 38,* 257-275.

Delamater, A. M., & Lahey, B. B. (1983). Physiological correlates of conduct disorder problems and anxiety in hyperactive and learning disabled children. *Journal of Abnormal Child Psychology, 11,* 85-100.

Delamater, A. M., Lahey, B. B., & Drake, L. (1981). Toward an empirical subclassification of "learning disabilities": A psychophysiological comparison of "hyperactive" and "non-hyperactive" subgroups. *Journal of Abnormal Child Psychology, 9,* 65-77.

Denkowski, K. M., Denkowski, G. C., & Omizo, M. M. (1983). The effects of EMG-assisted relaxation training on the academic performance, locus of control, and self-esteem of hyperactive boys. *Biofeedback and Self-Regulation, 8,* 363-375.

Douglas, V. I. (1975). Are drugs enough? To treat or train the hyperactive child. *International Journal of Mental Health, 4*, 199-212.

Douglas, V. I. (1980). Treatment and training approaches to hyperactivity: Establishing internal or external control. In C. K. Henker & B. Henker (Eds.), *Hyperactive children: The social ecology of identification and treatment.* New York: Academic Press.

Douglas, V. I., & Peters, K. G. (1979). Toward a clearer definition of the attentional deficit of hyperactive children. In G. A. Hale & M. Lewis (Eds.), *Attention and cognitive development.* New York: Plenum.

Douglas, V. I., Parry, P., Marton, P., & Gaston, C. (1976). Assessment of a cognitive training program for hyperactive children. *Journal of Abnormal Child Psychology, 4*, 389-410.

Duffy, F. H., Denckla, M. B., Bartels, P. H., & Sandini, G. (1980). Dyslexia: Regional differences in brain electrical activity by topographic mapping. *Annals of Neurology, 7*, 412-420.

Dunn, F. M., & Howell, R. J. (1982). Relaxation training and its relationship to hyperactivity in boys. *Journal of Clinical Psychology, 38*, 92-100.

Eastman, B. G., & Rasbury, W. C. (1981). Cognitive self-instruction for the control of impulsive classroom behavior: Ensuring the treatment package. *Journal of Abnormal Child Psychology, 9*, 381-387.

Eaton, W. O. (1983). Measuring activity level with actometers: Reliability, validity, and arm length. *Child Development, 54*, 720-726.

Edelbrock, C., & McLaughlin, B. (1980). Hierarchical cluster analysis using intraclass correlation: A mixture model study. *Multivariate Behavioral Research, 15*, 299-318.

Eisenberg, L., Conners, C. K., & Sharpe, L. (1965). A controlled study of the differential application of outpatient psychiatric treatment for children. *Japanese Journal of Child Psychiatry, 6*, 125-132.

Eisenberg, L., Gilbert, A., Cytryn, L., & Molling, P. (1961). The effectiveness of psychotherapy alone and in conjunction with perphenazine or placebo in the treatment of neurotic and hyperkinetic children. *American Journal of Psychiatry, 117*, 1088-1093.

Eisenberg, L., Lachman, R., Molling, P., Lockner, A., Mizelle, J., & Conners, C. K. (1963). A psychopharmacologic experiment in a training school for delinquent boys. *American Journal of Orthopsychiatry, 33*, 431-447.

Eysenck, H. J. (1952). *The scientific study of personality.* London: Routledge & Kegan Paul.

Eysenck, S.B.G., Easting, G., & Pearson, P. R. (1984). Age norms for impulsiveness, venturesomeness and empathy in children. *Personality and Individual Differences, 5*, 315-321.

Fedio, P., & Mirsky, A. F. (1969). Selective intellectual deficits in children with temporal lobe or centrencephalic epilepsy. *Neuropsychologia, 7*, 287-300.

Ferguson, H. B., & Rapoport, J. L. (1983). Nosological issues and biological validation. In M. Rutter (Ed.), *Developmental neuropsychiatry.* New York: Guilford.

Firestone, P. (1982). Factors associated with children's adherence to stimulant medication. *American Journal of Orthopsychiatry 52*, 447-457.

Firestone, P., Kelly, M. J., Goodman, J. T., & Davey, J. (1981). Differential effects of parent training and stimulant medication with hyperactives. *Journal of the American Academy of Child Psychiatry, 20*, 135-147.

Forehand, R., & McMahon, R. (1981). *Helping the noncompliant child: A clinician's guide to parent training.* New York: Guilford.

Forehand, R., Sturgis, E. T., McMahon, R. J., Aguar, D., Green, K., Wells, K. C., & Breiner, J. (1979). Parent behavioral training to modify child noncompliance: Treatment generalization across time and from home to school. *Behavior Modification, 3*, 3-25.

Friedling, C., & O'Leary, S. G. (1979). Effects of self-instructional training on second and third grade hyperactive children: A failure to replicate. *Journal of Applied Behavior Analysis, 12*, 211-219.

Frostig, M. (1961). *Developmental tasks of visual perception.* Palo Alto, CA: Consulting Psychologists Press.

Gadow, K. D. (1983). Effects of stimulant drugs on academic performance in hyperactive and learning disabled children. *Journal of Learning Disabilities, 16*, 290-296.

Gildea, M.C.L., Glidewell, J. C., & Kantor, M. B. (1961). Maternal attitudes and general adjustment in school children. In J. C. Glidewell (Ed.), *Parental attitudes and child behavior.* Springfield, Il: Charles C Thomas.

Gillberg, C., Carlstrom, G., & Rasmussen, P. (1983). Hyperkinetic disorders in seven-year-old children with perceptual, motor and attentional deficits. *Journal of Child Psychology and Psychiatry, 24*, 233-246.

Gittelman, R., Abikoff, H., Pollack, E., Klein, D., Katz, S., & Mattes, J. (1980). A controlled trial of behavior modification and methylphenidate in hyperactive children. In C. K. Whalen & B. Henker (Eds.), *Hyperactive children: The social ecology of identification and treatment*. New York: Academic Press.

Gittelman-Klein, R., & Klein, D. F. (1976). Methylphenidate effects in learning disabilities: Psychometric changes. *Archives of General Psychiatry, 33*, 655-664.

Gittelman-Klein, R., Klein, D. F., Abikoff, H., Katz, S., Gloisten, A. C., & Kates, W. (1976). Relative efficacy of methylphenidate and behavior modification in hyperkinetic children: An interim report. *Journal of Abnormal Child Psychology, 4*, 361-379.

Gorenstein, E. E., & Newman, J. P. (1980). Disinhibitory psychopathology: A new perspective and a model for research. *Psychological Bulletin, 87*, 301-315.

Gray, J. A. (1982). *The neuropsychology of anxiety: An enquiry into the functions of the septo-hippocampal system*. New York: Oxford University Press.

Guilford, J. P., & Zimmerman, S. (1956). Fourteen dimensions of temperament. *Psychological Monographs, 70* (Whole No. 417).

Guze, S. (1970). The need for tough-mindedness in psychiatric thinking. *Southern Medical Journal, 63*, 662-671.

Halverson, C. F., & Waldrop, M. F. (1973). The relations of mechanically recorded activity level to varieties of preschool play behavior. *Child Development, 44*, 678-681.

Harris, D. (1963). *Children's drawings as measures of intellectual maturity*. New York: Harcourt Brace & World.

Hastings, J. E., & Barkley, R. A. (1978). A review of psychophysiological research with hyperkinetic children. *Journal of Abnormal Child Psychology, 6*, 413-447.

Hebb, D. O. (1955). Drives and the CNS (conceptual nervous system). *Psychological Review, 62*, 243-252.

Hechtman, L., Weiss, G., Perlman, T., & Amsel, R. (1984). Hyperactives as young adults: Initial predictors of adult outcome. *American Academy of Child Psychiatry, 23*, 250-260.

Hicks, R. E., & Gualtieri, C. T. (unpublished). Differential psychopharmacology of methylphenidate and the neuropsychology of childhood hyperactivity. Department of Psychiatry and the Biological Sciences Research Center, University of North Carolina, Chapel Hill.

Hill, E. F. (1972). *The Holtzman inkblot technique*. San Francisco: Jossey-Bass.

Hillyard, S. A., Hink, R. F., Schwent, V. K., & Picton, T. W. (1973). Electrical signs of selective attention. *Science, 182*, 177-179.

Hinshaw, S. P., Henker, B., & Whalen, C. K. (1984). Self-control in hyperactive boys in anger-inducing situations: Effects of cognitive-behavioral training and of methylphenidate. *Journal of Abnormal Child Psychology, 12*, 55-77.

Hoffman, S. P., Engelhardt, D. M., Margolis, R. A., Polizos, P., Waizer, J., & Rosenfeld, R. (1974). Response to methylphenidate in low socioeconomic hyperactive children. *Archives of General Psychiatry, 30*, 354-359.

Holden, E., Tarnowski, K. J., & Prinz, R. J. (1982). Reliability of neurological soft signs in children: Reevaluation of the PANESS. *Journal of Abnormal Child Psychology, 10*, 163-172.

Holtzman, W. H. (1961). *Guide to administration and scoring: Holtzman inkblot technique*. New York: Psychological Corporation.

Holtzman, W. H., Thorpe, J. S., Swartz, J. D., & Herron, E. W. (1961). *Inkblot perception and personality*. Austin: University of Texas Press.

Horn, W. F., Chatoor, I., & Conners, C. K. (1983). Additive effects of dexedrine and self-control training: A multiple assessment. *Behavior Modification, 7*, 383-402.

Humphries, T., Kinsbourne, M., & Swanson, J. (1978). Stimulant effects on cooperation and social interaction between hyperactive children and their mothers. *Journal of Child Psychology and Psychiatry, 19*, 13-22.

Humphries, T., Swanson, J. M., Kinsbourne, M., & Yiu, L. (1979). Stimulant effects on persistence of motor performance of hyperactive children. *Journal of Pediatric Psychology, 4*, 55-66.

Hutt, S. J., & Hutt, C. (1970). *Direct observation and measurement of behavior*. Springfield, Il: Charles C Thomas.

Jastak, J. F., & Jastak, S. R. (1965). *The Wide Range Achievement Test*. Wilmington: Guidance Associates.

Johnson, C. F. (1971). Hyperactivity and the machine: The actometer. *Child Development, 42*, 2105-2110.

Jouandet, M., & Gazzaniga, M. S. (1979). The frontal lobes. In M. Gazzaniga (Ed.), *Handbook of behavioral neurobiology* (Vol. 2). New York: Plenum.

Kahneman, D. (1973). *Attention and effort.* Englewood Cliffs, NJ: Prentice-Hall.

Kaufman, A. S. (1979). *Intelligent testing with the WISC-R.* New York: Wiley.

Kendall, P. C., & Brophy, C. (1981). Activity and attentional correlates of teacher ratings of hyperactivity. *Journal of Pediatric Psychology, 6,* 451-458.

Kenny, T. J. (1980). Hyperactivity. In H. E. Rie & E. D. Rie (Eds.), *Handbook of minimal brain dysfunctions: A critical view.* New York: Wiley.

Kenny, T. J., Clemmens, R. L., Hudson, B. W., Lentz, G. A., Cicci, R., & Nair, P. (1971). Characteristics of children referred because of hyperactivity. *Journal of Pediatrics, 79,* 618-622.

Kershner, J. R., & King, A. J. (1974). Laterality of cognitive functions in achieving hemiplegic children. *Perceptual and Motor Skills, 39,* 1283-1289.

Kessler, J. W. (1980). History of minimal brain dysfunction. In H. E. Rie & E. D. Rie (Eds.), *Handbook of minimal brain dysfunctions: A critical view.* New York: Wiley.

Kinsbourne, M. (1973). Minimal brain dysfunction as a neurodevelopmental lag. *Annals of The New York Academy of Sciences, 205,* 263-273.

Kinsbourne, M. (1979). Models of hyperactivity: Implications for diagnosis and treatment. In R. L. Trites (Ed.), *Hyperactivity in children: Etiology, measurement, and treatment implications.* Baltimore: University Park Press.

Klein, D. F., Gittelman, R., Quitkin, F., & Rifkin, A. (1980). *Diagnosis and drug treatment of psychiatric disorders: Adults and children* (2nd ed.). Baltimore: Williams & Wilkins.

Klorman, R., Salzman, L. F., Pass, H. L., Borgstedt, A. D., & Dainer, K. B. (1979). Effects of methylphenidate on hyperactive children's evoked responses during passive and active attention. *Psychophysiology, 16,* 23-29.

Klove, H., & Hole, K. (1979). The hyperkinetic syndrome: Criteria for diagnosis. In R. L. Trites (Ed.), *Hyperactivity in children: Etiology, measurement and treatment implications.* Baltimore: University Park Press.

Koppitz, E. (1964). *Bender Gestalt test for young children.* New York: Grune & Stratton.

Lahey, B. B., Stempniak, M., Robinson, E. J., & Tyroler, M. J. (1978). Hyperactivity and learning disabilities as independent dimensions of child behavior problems. *Journal of Abnormal Psychology, 87,* 333-340.

Lambert, N. M., & Hartsough, C. S. (1984). Contribution of predispositional factors to the diagnosis of hyperactivity. *American Journal of Orthopsychiatry, 54,* 97-109.

Lambert, N. M., Sandoval, J., & Sassone, D. (1978). Prevalence of hyperactivity in elementary school children as a function of the social system definers. *American Journal of Orthopsychiatry, 48,* 446-463.

Landis, C., & Hunt, W. A. (1939). *The startle pattern.* New York: Farrar & Rinehart.

Lang, P. J., Ohman, A., & Simons, R. F. (1978). The psychophysiology of anticipation. In J. Requin (Ed.), *Attention and performance* (Vol. 7), Hillsdale, NJ: Lawrence Erlbaum.

Langhorne, J. E., Jr., Loney, J., Paternite, C. E., & Bechtoldt, H. P. (1976). Childhood hyperkinesis: A return to the source. *Journal of Abnormal Psychology, 85,* 201-209.

Larsen, B., Skinhoj, E., & Lassen, N. A. (1978). Variations in regional cortical blood flow in the right and left hemispheres during automatic speech. *Brain, 101,* 193-210.

Lassen, N. A., Ingvar, D. H., & Skinhoj, E. (1978). Brain function and blood flow. *Scientific American, 239,* 62-71.

Laufer, M. W., & Denhoff, E. (1957). Hyperkinetic impulse disorder in children. *Journal of Pediatrics, 50,* 463-474.

Levy, F. (1980). The development of sustained attention (vigilance) and inhibition in children: Some normative data. *Journal of Child Psychology and Psychiatry, 21,* 77-84.

Loiselle, D. L., Stamm, J. S., Maitinsky, S., & Whipple, S. C. (1980). Evoked potential and behavioral signs of attentive dysfunctions in hyperactive boys. *Psychophysiology, 17,* 193-201.

Loney, J., Weissenburger, F. E., Woolson, R. F., & Lichty, E. C. (1979). Comparing psychological and pharmocological treatments for hyperkinetic boys and their classmates. *Journal of Abnormal Child Psychology, 7,* 133-143.

Lou, H. C., Henriksen, L., & Bruhn, P. (1984). Focal cerebral hypoperfusion in children with dysphasia and/or attention deficit disorder. *Archives of Neurology, 41,* 825-829.

Lovrich, D., & Stamm, J. S. (1983). Event-related potential and behavior correlates of attention in reading retardation. *Journal of Clinical Neuropsychology, 5,* 13-37.

Lucas, A. R. (1980). Muscular control and coordination in minimal brain dysfunction. In H. E. Rie & E. D. Rie (Eds.), *Handbook of minimal brain dysfunctions: A critical view.* New York: Wiley.

Luria, A. R. (1960). *The nature of human conflicts: An objective study of disorganization and control of human behaviour.* New York: Grove Press.

Luria, A., & Yudovich, F. (1959). *Speech and the development of mental processes in the child.* New York: Staples.

MacLean, P. D. (1949). Psychosomatic disease and the "visceral brain": Recent developments bearing on the Papez theory of emotion. *Psychosomatic Medicine, 11,* 338-353.

Mash, E. J., & Johnston C. (1983). The prediction of mothers' behavior with their hyperactive children during play and task situations. *Child and Family Behavior Therapy, 5,* 1-14.

Mattes, J. A. (1980). The role of frontal lobe dysfunction in childhood hyperkinesis. *Comprehensive Psychiatry, 21,* 358-368.

Meichenbaum, D. H., & Goodman, J. (1971). Training impulsive children to talk to themselves: A means of developing self-control. *Journal of Abnormal Psychology, 77,* 115-126.

Mercier, L., & Pivik, R. T. (1983). Spinal motoneuronal excitability during wakefulness and non-REM sleep in hyperkinesis. *Journal of Clinical Neuropsychology, 5,* 321-336.

Michael, R. L., Klorman, R., Salzman, L. F., Borgstedt, A. D., & Dainer, K. B. (1981). Normalizing effects of methylphenidate on hyperactive children's vigilance performance and evoked potentials. *Psychophysiology, 18,* 665-677.

Mikkelsen, E. J., Brown, G. L., Minichiello, M. D., Millican, F. K., & Rapoport, J. L. (1982). Neurologic status in hyperactive, enuretic, encopretic and normal boys. *Journal of the American Academy of Child Psychiatry, 21,* 75-81.

Milich, R. (1984). Cross-sectional and longitudinal observations of activity level and sustained attention in a normative sample. *Journal of Abnormal Child Psychology, 12,* 261-276.

Milich, R. S., & Loney, J. (1979). The role of hyperactive and aggressive symptomatology in predicting adolescent outcome among hyperactive children. *Journal of Pediatric Psychology, 4,* 93-112.

Millichap, J. G., & Boldrey, E. E. (1967). Studies in hyperkinetic behavior. II. Laboratory and clinical evaluation of drug treatments. *Neurology, 17,* 467-474.

Morrison, J. R., & Stewart, M. A. (1971). A family study of the hyperactive child syndrome. *Biological Psychiatry, 3,* 189-195.

Naatanen, R. (1970). Evoked potential, EEG and slow potential correlates of selective attention. *Acta Psychologica, 33,* 178-192.

Naatanen, R. (1982). Processing negativity: An evoked-potential reflection of selective attention. *Psychological Bulletin, 92,* 605-640.

Naatanen, R., Simpson, M., & Loveless, N. E. (1982). Stimulus deviance versus significance and event-related brain potentials. *Biological Psychology, 14,* 53-98.

Nauta, W.J.H. (1971). The problem of the frontal lobe: A reinterpretation. *Journal of Psychiatric Research, 8,* 167-187.

Nebylitsyn, V. D. (1972). *Fundamental properties of the human nervous system.* New York: Plenum.

O'Gorman, J. G. (1977). Individual differences in habituation of human physiological responses: A review of theory, method, and findings in the study of personality correlates in nonclinical populations. *Biological Psychiatry, 5,* 257-318.

O'Leary, K. D., & O'Leary, S. G. (1977). *Classroom management: The successful use of behavior modification* (2nd ed.). Elmsford, NY: Pergamon.

O'Leary, K. D., Pelham, W. E., Rosenbaum, A., & Price, G. H. (1976). Behavioral treatment of hyperkinetic children: An experimental evalution of its usefulness. *Clinical Pediatrics, 15,* 510-515.

Omizo, M. M., & Michael, W. B. (1982). Biofeedback-induced relaxation training and impulsivity, attention to task, and locus of control among hyperactive boys. *Journal of Learning Disabilities, 15,* 414-416.

Owen, D., & Sines, J. O. (1970). Heritability of personality in children. *Behavior Genetics, 1,* 235-248.

Paternite, C. E., & Loney, J. (1980). Childhood hyperkinesis: Relationships between symptomatology and home environment. In C. K. Whalen & B. Henker (Eds.), *Hyperactive children: The social ecology of identification and treatment.* New York: Academic Press.

Paternite, C. E., Loney, J., & Langhorne, J. E. (1976). Relationships between symptomatology and SES-related factors in hyperkinetic/MBD boys. *American Journal of Orthopsychiatry, 46*, 291-301.

Patterson, G. R. (1983). *Coercive family process.* Eugene, OR: Castalia.

Peeke, S., Halliday, R., Callaway, E., Prael, R., & Reus, V. (1984). Effects of two doses of methylphenidate on verbal information processing in hyperactive children. *Journal of Clinical Psychopharmacology, 4*, 82-88.

Pelham, W. (1983). The effects of psychostimulants on academic achievement in hyperactive and learning-disabled children. *Thalamus, 3*, 1-48.

Pelham, W. E., & Murphy, H. A. (1985). *Behavioral and pharmacological treatment of attention deficit and conduct disorders.* Unpublished manuscript.

Pelham, W. E., Schnedler, R. W., Bender, M. E., Nillson, D. E., Miller, J., Budrow, M. S., Ronnei, M., Paluchowski, C., & Marks, D. (1985). The combination of behavior therapy and methylphenidate in the treatment of attention deficit disorders: A therapy outcome study. In L. Bloomingdale (Ed.), *Attention deficit disorders* (Vol. 3). New York: Spectrum.

Pelham, W., Schnedler, R., Bologna, N., & Contreras, A. (1980). Behavioral and stimulant treatment of hyperactive children: A therapy study with methylphenidate probes in a within-subject design. *Journal of Applied Behavior Analysis, 13*, 221-236.

Peterson, D. R. (1961). Behavior problems of middle childhood. *Journal of Consulting Psychology, 25*, 205-209.

Pfadt, A., & Tryon, W. W. (1983). Issues in the selection and use of mechanical transducers to directly measure motor activity in clinical settings. *Applied Research in Mental Retardation, 4*, 251-270.

Picton, T. W., Campbell, K. B., Baribeau-Braun, J., & Prouix, G. B. (1978). The neurophysiology of human attention: A tutorial review. In J. Requin (Ed.), *Attention and performance* (Vol. 7). Hillsdale, NJ: Erlbaum.

Pivik, R. T., & Mercier, L. (1979). Motoneuronal excitability during wakefulness and non-REM sleep: H-reflex recovery function in man. *Sleep, 1*, 357-367.

Pollard, S., Ward, E. M., & Barkley, R. A. (1983). The effects of parent training and Ritalin on the parent-child interactions of hyperactive boys. *Child and Family Behavior Therapy, 5*, 51-69.

Pontius, A. (1973). Dysfunction patterns analogous to frontal lobe system and caudate nucleus syndromes in some groups of minimal brain dysfunction. *Journal of the American Medical Women's Association, 28*, 285-212.

Pope, L. (1970). Motor activity in brain injured children. *American Journal of Orthopsychiatry, 40*, 783-794.

Porges, S. W. (1976). Peripheral and neurochemical parallels of psychopathology: A psychophysiological model relating autonomic imbalance to hyperactivity, psychopathy and autism. In H. W. Reese (Ed.), *Advances in child development and behavior* (Vol. 11).

Porges, S. W., & Smith, K. M. (1980). Defining hyperactivity: Psychophysiological and behavioral strategies. In C. K. Whalen & B. Henker (Eds.), *Hyperactive children: The social ecology of identification and treatment.* New York: Academic Press.

Porges, S. W., Walter, G. F., Korb, R. J., & Sprague, R. L. (1975). The influence of methylphenidate on heart rate and behavioral measures of attention in hyperactive children. *Child Development, 46*, 727-733.

Porrino, L. J., Rapoport, J. L., Behar, D., Sceery, W., Ismond, D. R., & Bunney, W. E., Jr. (1983). A naturalistic assessment of the motor activity of hyperactive boys. *Archives of General Psychiatry, 40*, 681-687.

Porteus, S. D. (1959). *The maze test and clinical psychology.* Palo Alto, CA: Pacific Books.

Porteus, S. D. (1965). *Porteus Maze Tests: Fifty years application.* Palo Alto, CA: Pacific Books.

Posner, M. I. (1975). Psychobiology of attention. In M. S. Gazzaniga & C. Blakemore (Eds.), *Handbook of psychobiology.* New York: Academic Press.

Quay, H. C. (1979). Classification. In H. C. Quay & J. S. Werry (Eds.), *Psychopathological disorders of childhood* (2nd ed.). New York: Wiley.

Quay, H. C. (in press). The behavioral reward and inhibition system in childhood behavior disorder. In L. M. Bloomingdale (Ed.), *Attention deficit disorder* (Vol. 3). New York: Spectrum.

Rapoport, J. L., Buchsbaum, M. S., Weingartner, H., Zahn, T. P., Ludlow, C., & Mikkelsen, E. J. (1980). Dextroamphetamine: Its cognitive and behavioral effects in normal and hyperactive boys and normal men. *Archives of General Psychiatry, 37*, 933-943.

Rapoport, J. L., Buchsbaum, M. S., Zahn, T. P., Weingartner, H., Ludlow, C., & Mikkelsen, E. J. (1978). Dextroamphetamine: Cognitive and behavioral effects in normal prepubertal boys. *Science, 199,* 560-563.

Requin, J. (1969). Some data on neurophysiological processes involved in the preparatory motor activity to reaction performance. *Acta Psychologica, 30,* 358-367.

Riddle, K. D., & Rapoport, J. L. (1976). A 2-year follow-up of 72 hyperactive boys. *Journal of Nervous and Mental Disease, 162,* 126-134.

Rie, E. D. (1980). Effects of MBD on learning, intellective functions, and achievement. In H. E. Rie & E. D. Rie (Eds.), *Handbook of minimal brain dysfunctions: A critical view.* New York: Wiley.

Robins, E., & Guze, S. (1970). Establishment of diagnostic validity and psychiatric illness: Its application to schizophrenia. *American Journal of Psychiatry, 126,* 983-987.

Robins, L. N. (1979). Follow-up studies. In H. C. Quay & J. S. Werry (Eds.), *Psychopathological disorders of childhood* (2nd ed.). New York: Wiley.

Rosenbaum, A., O'Leary, K. D., & Jacob, R. G. (1975). Behavioral intervention with hyperactive children: Group consequences as a supplement to individual contingencies. *Behavior Therapy, 6,* 315-323.

Ross, D. M., & Ross, S. A. (1982). *Hyperactivity: Current issues, research and theory* (2nd ed.). New York: Wiley.

Rourke, B. P., & Telegdy, G. A. (1971). Lateralizing significance of WISC Verbal-Performance discrepancies for older children with learning disabilities. *Perceptual and Motor Skills, 33,* 875-883.

Rourke, B. P., Bakker, D. J., Fisk, J. L., & Strang, J. D. (1983). *Child neuropsychology: An introduction to theory, research, and clinical practice.* New York: Guilford.

Routh, D. K., & Roberts, R. D. (1972). Minimal brain dysfunction in children: Failure to find evidence for a behavioral syndrome. *Psychological Reports, 31,* 307-314.

Routh, D. S., & Schroeder, C. S. (1976). Standardized playroom measures as indices of hyperactivity. *Journal of Abnormal Child Psychology, 4,* 199-207.

Routh, D., Schroeder, C., & O'Tuama, L. (1974). Development of activity level in children. *Developmental Psychology, 10,* 163-168.

Rudel, R. (1982). The oblique mystique. A slant on the development of spatial coordinates. In M. Potegal (Ed.), *Spatial abilities: Development and physiological foundations.* New York: Academic Press.

Rudel, R., & Teuber, H. L. (1971). Spatial orientation in normal children and in children with early brain injury. *Neuropsychologia, 9,* 401-407.

Rudel, R., Teuber, H. L., & Twitchell, T. E. (1974). Levels of impairment of sensorimotor functions in children with early brain damage. *Neuropsychologica 12,* 95-108.

Rutter, M. (1982). Syndromes attributed to "minimal brain dysfunction" in childhood. *American Journal of Psychiatry, 139,* 21-33.

Rutter, M. (1983). Behavioral studies: Questions and findings on the concept of a distinctive syndrome. In M. Rutter (Ed.), *Developmental neuropsychiatry.* New York: Guilford.

Rutter, M., & Graham, P. (1968). The reliability and validity of the psychiatric assessment of the child: I. Interview with the child. *British Journal of Psychiatry, 114,* 563-579.

Rutter, M., Graham, P., & Yule, W. (1970). A neuropsychiatric study in childhood. *Clinics in Developmental Medicine Nos. 35-36.* London: Heinemann Medical Books.

Rutter, M., Shaffer, D., & Shepherd, M. (1975). *A multiaxial classification of child psychiatric disorders.* Geneva: World Health Organization.

Safer, D. J., & Allen, R. P. (1976). *Hyperactive children: Diagnosis and management.* Baltimore: University Park Press.

Sandberg, S., Weiselberg, M., & Shaffer, D. (1980). Hyperkinetic and conduct problem children in a primary school population: Some epidemiological considerations. *Journal of Child Psychology and Psychiatry, 21,* 293-311.

Sandberg, S. T., Rutter, M., & Taylor, E. (1978). Hyperkinetic disorder in psychiatric clinic attenders. *Developmental Medicine and Child Neurology, 20,* 279-299.

Satterfield, J. H., & Braley, B. W. (1977). Evoked potentials and brain maturation in hyperactive children. *Electroencephalography and Clinical Neurophysiology, 43,* 43-51.

Satterfield, J. H., Cantwell, D., & Satterfield, B. (1974). Pathophysiology of the hyperactive child syndrome. *Archives of General Psychiatry, 31,* 839-844.

Satterfield, J. H., Cantwell, D. P., & Satterfield, B. T. (1979). Multimodality treatment. *Archives of General Psychiatry, 36*, 965-974.

Satterfield, J. H., Satterfield, B. T., & Cantwell, D. P. (1980). Multimodality treatment: A two-year evaluation of 61 hyperactive boys. *Archives of General Psychiatry, 37*, 915-918.

Satterfield, J. H., Satterfield, B. T., & Cantwell, D. P. (1981). Three-year multi-modality treatment study of 100 hyperactive boys. *Journal of Pediatrics, 98*, 650-655.

Satterfield, J. H., & Schell, A. M. (1984). Childhood brain function differences in delinquent and non-delinquent hyperactive boys. *Electroencephalography and Clinical Neurophysiology, 57*, 199-207.

Scarr, S. (1966). Genetic factors in activity motivation. *Child Development, 37*, 663-673.

Scheibel, M. E., & Scheibel, A. B. (1967). Anatomical basis of attention mechanisms in vertebrate brains. In G. C. Quarton, T. Melnechuk, & F. O. Schmitt (Eds.), *The neurosciences: A study program*. New York: Rockefeller University Press.

Schellekens, J.M.H., Scholten, C. A., & Kalverboer, A. F. (1983). Visually guided hand movements in children with minor neurological dysfunction: Response time and movement organization. *Journal of Child Psychiatry and Psychology, 24*, 89-102.

Schoenfeldt, L. F. (1968). The hereditary components of the Project TALENT two-day test battery. *Measurement and Evaluation in Guidance, 1*, 130-140.

Schulman, J. L., & Reisman, J. M. (1959). An objective measure of hyperactivity. *American Journal of Mental Deficiency, 64*, 455-456.

Sergeant, J. A., & Scholten, C. A. (1983). A stages-of-information approach to hyperactivity. *Journal of Child Psychology and Psychiatry, 24*, 49-60.

Shafer, S. Q., Shaffer, D., O'Connor, P. A., & Stokman, C. J. (1983). Hard thoughts on neurological "soft signs." In M. Rutter (Ed.), *Developmental neuropsychiatry*. New York: Guilford.

Shaffer, D., & Greenhill, L. (1979). A critical note on the predictive validity of "the hyperkinetic syndrome." *Journal of Child Psychology and Psychiatry, 20*, 61-72.

Shaffer, D., O'Connor, P. A., Shafer, S. Q., & Prupis, S. (1983). Neurological "soft signs": Their origins and significance. In M. Rutter (Ed.), *Developmental neuropsychiatry*. New York: Guilford.

Shaywitz, S. E., Shaywitz, B. A., Cohen, D. J., & Young, J. G. (1983). Monoaminergic mechanisms in hyperactivity. In M. Rutter (Ed.), *Developmental neuropsychiatry*. New York: Guilford.

Shih, T. M., Khachaturian, Z. S., Barry, H., III, & Reisler, K. L. (1975). Differential effects of methylphenidate on reticular formation and thalamic neuronal activity. *Psychopharmacologia, 44*, 11-15.

Siddle, D.A.T., & Mangan, G. L. (1971). Arousability and individual differences in resistance to distraction. *Journal of Experimental Research in Personality, 5*, 295-303.

Skinner, J. E., & Yingling, C. D. (1977). Central gating mechanisms that regulate event-related potentials and behavior: A neural model for attention. In J. E. Desmedt (Ed.), *Progress in neurophysiology. Vol. 1: Attention, voluntary contraction and event-related cerebral potentials*. Basel: Karger.

Snyder, E., & Hillyard, S. A. (1976). Long latency evoked potential to irrelevant deviant stimuli. *Behavioral Biology, 16*, 319-331.

Sokolov, E. N. (1969). The modelling properties of the nervous system. In M. Cole & I. Maltzman (Eds.), *Handbook of contemporary Soviet psychology*. London: Basic Books.

Solanto, M. V., & Conners, C. K. (1982). A dose-response and time-action analysis of autonomic and behavior effects of methylphenidate in attention deficit disorder with hyperactivity. *Psychophysiology, 19*, 657-658.

Sprague, R. L., & Sleator, E. K. (1976). Drugs and dosages: Implications for learning disabilities. In R. M. Knights & D. J. Bakker (Eds.), *Neuropsychology of learning disorders: Theoretical approaches*. Baltimore: University Park Press.

Sprague, R. L., & Sleator, E. K. (1977). Methylphenidate in hyperkinetic children: Differences in dose effects on learning and social behavior. *Science, 198*, 1274-1276.

Sroufe, L. A. (1975). Drug treatment of children with behavior problems. In F. D. Horowitz (Ed.), *Review of child development research* (Vol. 4). Chicago: University of Chicago Press.

Sroufe, L. A., Sonies, B. C., West, W. D., & Wright, F. S. (1973). Anticipatory heart rate deceleration and reaction time in children with and without referral for learning disability. *Child Development, 44*, 267-273.

Stamm, J. S., & Kreder, S. V. (1979). Minimal brain dysfunction: Psychological and neurophysiological disorders in hyperkinetic children. In M. S. Gazzaniga (Ed.), *Handbook of behavioral neurobiology* (Vol. 2). New York: Plenum.

Stevens, T. M., Kupst, M. J., Suran, B. G., & Schulman, J. L. (1978). Activity level: a comparison between actometer scores and observer ratings. *Journal of Abnormal Child Psychology, 6*, 163-173.

Sykes, D. H., Douglas, V. I., & Morgenstern, G. (1973). Sustained attention in hyperactive children. *Journal of Child Psychology and Psychiatry, 14*, 213-220.

Taylor, E. (1983). Drug response and diagnostic validation. In M. Rutter (Ed.), *Developmental neuropsychiatry*. New York: Guilford.

Thomas, A., & Chess, S. (1977). *Temperament and development*. New York: Brunner/Mazel.

Thurstone, L. L. (1951). The dimensions of temperament. *Psychometrika, 16*, 11-20.

Trites, R. L., & Laprade, K. (1983). Evidence for an independent syndrome of hyperactivity. *Journal of Child Psychiatry and Psychology, 24*, 573-586.

Waters, W. F., McDonald, D. G., & Koresko, R. L. (1977). Habituation of the orienting response: A gating mechanism subserving selective attention. *Psychophysiology, 14*, 228-236.

Webb, R. A., & Obrist, P. S. (1970). The physiological concomitants of reaction time performance as a function of preparatory interval and preparatory interval series. *Psychophysiology, 6*, 389-403.

Wechsler, D. (1949). *Wechsler Intelligence Scale for Children*. New York: Psychological Corporation.

Weiss, G., Hechtman, L., Perlman, T., Hopkins, J., & Wener, A. (1979). Hyperactive children as young adults: A controlled prospective 10 year follow-up of the psychiatric status of 75 hyperactive children. *Archives of General Psychiatry, 36*, 675-681.

Weiss, G., Kruger, E., Danielson, U., & Elman, M. (1975). Effects of long-term treatment of hyperactive children with methylphenidate. *Canadian Medical Association Journal, 112*, 159-165.

Weiss, G., Minde, K., Werry, J. S., Douglas, V. I., & Nemeth, E. (1971). Studies on the hyperactive child, VIII: Five-year follow-up. *Archives of General Psychiatry, 24*, 409-414.

Wells, K. C., Conners, C. K., Imber, L., & Delamater, A. (1981). Use of single-subject methodology in clinical decision-making with a hyperactive child on the psychiatric inpatient unit. *Behavioral Assessment, 3*, 359-369.

Wells, K. C., & Forehand, R. (1981). Childhood behavior problems in the home. In S. M. Turner, K. S. Calhoun, & H. E. Adams (Eds.), *Handbook of clinical behavior therapy*. New York: Wiley.

Wells, K. C., & Forehand, R. (1985). Conduct and oppositional disorders. In P. H. Bornstein & A. E. Kazdin (Eds.), *Handbook of clinical behavior therapy with children*. New York: Dorsey Press.

Werner, E. E. (1980). Environmental interaction in minimal brain dysfunctions. In H. E. Rie & E. D. Rie (Eds.), *Handbook of minimal brain dysfunctions: A critical view*. New York: Wiley.

Werry, J. S. (1968). Studies on the hyperactive child, IV. An empirical analysis of the minimal brain dysfunction syndrome. *Archives of General Psychiatry, 19*, 9-16.

Werry, J. S. (1978). *Pediatric psychopharmacology: The use of behavior modifying drugs in children*. New York: Brunner/Mazel.

Werry, J. S. (1979). Organic factors. In H. C. Quay & J. S. Werry (Eds.), *Psychopathological disorders of childhood* (2nd ed.). New York: Wiley.

Werry, J. S., Minde, K., Guzman, A., Weiss, G., Dogan, K., & Hoy, E. (1972). Studies on the hyperactive child: VII. Neurological status compared with neurotic and normal children. *American Journal of Orthopsychiatry, 42*, 441-451.

Werry, J. S., Weiss, G., Douglas, V., & Martin, J. (1966). Studies on the hyperactive child: III. The effect of chlorpromazine upon behavior and learning ability. *Journal of the American Academy of Child Psychiatry, 5*, 292-312.

Whalen, C. K. (1983). Hyperactivity, learning problems, and the attention deficit disorders. In T. H. Ollendick & M. Hersen (Eds.), *Handbook of child psychopathology*. New York: Plenum.

Whalen, C. K., Collins, B. E., Henker, B., Alkus, S. R., Adams, D., & Stapp, J. (1978). Behavior observations of hyperactive children and methylphenidate (Ritalin) effects in systematically structured classroom environments. *Journal of Pediatric Psychology, 3*, 177-184.

Whalen, C. K., & Henker, B. (1976). Psychostimulants and children: A review and analysis. *Psychological Bulletin, 83*, 1113-1130.

Whalen, C. K., & Henker, B. (1977). The pitfalls of politicization. A response to Conrad's "The discovery of hyperkinesis": Notes on the medicalization of deviant behavior. *Social Problems, 24*, 590-595.

Whalen, C. K., & Henker, B. (1980a). The social ecology of psychostimulant treatment: A model for conceptual and empirical analysis. In C. K. Whalen & B. Henker (Eds.), *Hyperactive children: The social ecology of identification and treatment*. New York: Academic Press.

Whalen, C. K., & Henker, B. (Eds.) (1980b). *Hyperactive children: The social ecology of identification and treatment*. New York: Academic Press.

Whalen, C. K., Henker, B., Collins, B. E., Finck, D., & Dotemoto, S. (1979a). A social ecology of hyperactive boys: Medication effects in structured classroom environments. *Journal of Applied Behavior Analysis, 12*, 65-81.

Whalen, C. K., Henker, B., Collins, B. E., McAuliffe, S., & Vaux, A. (1979b). Peer interaction in a structured communication task: Comparisons of normal and hyperactive boys and of methylphenidate (Ritalin) and placebo effects. *Child Development, 50*, 388-401.

Whalen, C. K., Henker, B., & Dotemoto, S. (1980). Methylphenidate and hyperactivity: Effects on teacher behaviors. *Science, 208*, 1280-1282.

Whalen, C. K., Henker, B., & Dotemoto, S. (1981). Teacher response to the methylphenidate (Ritalin) versus placebo status of hyperactive boys in the classroom. *Child Development, 52*, 1005-1014.

Whalen, C. K., Henker, B., & Finck, D. (1981). Medication effects in the classroom: Three naturalistic indicators. *Journal of Abnormal Child Psychology, 9*, 419-433.

Wilkinson, R. T., & Lee, M. V. (1972). Auditory evoked potentials and selective attention. *EEG and Clinical Neurophysiology, 33*, 411-418.

Willerman, L. (1973). Activity level and hyperactivity in twins. *Child Development, 44*, 288-293.

Wolraich, M. L., Drummond, T., Saloman, M. K., O'Brien, M. L., & Sivage, C. (1978). Effects of methylphenidate alone and in combination with behavior modification procedures on the behavior and academic performance of hyperactive children. *Journal of Abnormal Child Psychology, 6*, 149-161.

Woods, B. T., & Eby, M. D. (1982). Excessive mirror movements and aggression. *Biological Psychiatry, 17*, 23-32.

Yakovlev, P. I., & Lecours, A. R. (1967). The myelogenetic cycles of regional maturation of the brain. In A. Minkowski (Ed.), *Regional development of the brain in early life*. Oxford: Blackwell.

Yingling, C. D., & Skinner, J. E. (1976). Selective regulation of thalamic sensory relay nuclei by nucleus reticularis thalami. *Electroencephalography and Clinical Neurophysiology, 41*, 476-482.

Zahn, T. P., Abate, F., Little, B. C., & Wender, P. H. (1975). Minimal brain dysfunction, stimulant drugs and autonomic nervous system activity. *Archives of General Psychiatry, 32*, 381-387.

Zambelli, A. J., Stamm, J. S., Maitinsky, S., & Loiselle, D. L. (1977). Auditory evoked potentials and selective attention in formerly hyperactive adolescents. *American Journal of Psychiatry, 134*, 742-747.

Zentall, S. S., & Zentall, T. R. (1983). Optimal stimulation: A model of disordered activity and performance in normal and deviant children. *Psychological Bulletin, 94*, 446-471.

INDEX

ABOUT THE AUTHORS

C. Keith Conners, Ph.D., received his undergraduate training at the University of Chicago. He was a Rhodes Scholar at Oxford, receiving First Class Honors in the School of Psychology, Philosophy, and Physiology. He received his Ph.D. from Harvard University in clinical psychology. He has taught at Johns Hopkins Medical School, Harvard University Medical School, and the University of Pittsburgh Medical School. He is currently Professor of Psychiatry at George Washington University Medical School, and Research Professor of Neurology at Children's Hospital National Medical Center, where he is also director of the Laboratory of Behavioral Medicine.

Karen C. Wells, Ph.D., attended undergraduate school at the University of Georgia, where she also received her Ph.D. in clinical psychology. She has taught at the University of Pittsburgh Medical School and is currently Associate Professor of Psychiatry at George Washington University Medical School, and Associate Professor of Child Health and Development at Children's Hospital National Medical Center in Washington, D.C.